Praise for Margit Novack's *Squint*

"This positive, affirming book will inspire and guide people as they navigate the third age of life. At once both profound and comforting, Novack's stories are as memorable as they are wise."
–KEN DYCHTWALD, PH.D., author of *What Retirees Want: A Holistic View of Life's Third Age* and *Radical Curiosity: One Man's Search for Cosmic Magic and a Purposeful Life*

"This book is a well-written, thoughtfully crafted exploration of many aspects of aging. The wisdom shared and insights offered provide a delightful and poignant journey through the common experiences of the second half of life, including caregiving, creating a legacy, and changing relationships and roles. Well worth the read!"
–TEEPA SNOW, Occupational Therapist and CEO of Positive Approach to Care®

"Too many Americans don't want to think about getting older, let alone look it in the eye. *Squint*, Margit Novack's illuminating memoir, offers a wise and welcome alternative. Novack writes with grace about the hard stuff, the funny stuff, the complicated stuff—hell, it's *all* complicated—and leaves her readers far better equipped for the years ahead."
–ASHTON APPLEWHITE, author of *This Chair Rocks: A Manifesto Against Ageism*

"Reflecting on her career as a Senior Move Manager, Margit Novack concludes that the objects we possess and let go have their real value as vessels for stories, even the difficult ones. As imperfect and impermanent as human lives are, the world will be better, she writes, for our passing those stories on."
–DAVID J. EKERDT, PH.D., Sociologist and Gerontologist, University of Kansas

"Margit Novack's delightful memoir, *Squint: Re-visioning the Second Half of Life*, opens our eyes wide to the abundant possibilities of later life. She pairs fascinating personal stories with larger themes (downsizing, caregiving, forgiveness, estrangement, and more) to help us navigate the uneven terrain of aging. She generously offers her rich cache of memories as the treasures they are—not unlike the precious possessions of her many senior move clients through the years. Margit skillfully weaves the impactful people and events of her own 70-something life, with need-to-know information about aging and retirement for everyone. I couldn't put it down, so I recommend you pick it up. I hope Volume II is already in the works. When you meet Bubbie and Anya, you will, too."
–MARY KAY BUYSSE, Executive Director, National Association of Senior & Specialty Move Managers

"*Squint: Re-Visioning the Second Half of Life* is about all of us and our own aging process, told masterfully through personal stories and solutions by author Margit Novack in her compelling, must-read book.

If we want to understand how once we reach mid-life, moving forward is more important than looking backward, get ready to take notes. This book covers it all—from loss, to learning something new, staying current with technology, becoming a caregiver with insights and tricks, the importance of being needed, getting rid of sibling estrangements, cleverly dividing family treasures, downsizing and determining the legacy you want to leave."

–VICKI THOMAS, Chief Purpose Officer, My Future Purpose

"One of the most powerful ways to learn is through story telling. Margit Novack, author of *Squint: Re-Visioning the Second Half of Life*, has mastered the art. As a pioneer in the move management industry, Novack examines her life and shares her personal stories that combine her experience, knowledge, resilience and insight sprinkled with humor to deliver profound and memorable messages about aging and the potential for growth and possibilities. This book is a gift that is realistic, compassionate, substantive and uplifting—telling it straight about aging and more. It's a must read . . . and must have for an enlightening and joyful journey."

–HELEN DENNIS, Columnist, Author and Specialist on Aging and the New Retirement

Squint

Squint

*Re-visioning the
Second Half of Life*

Margit Novack

Extra Step Media

Cover design by Tabitha Lahr
Interior text design by Tabitha Lahr
Title page illustration © Shutterstock.com

978-0-578-93303-0 (print)
978-0-578-93304-7 (eBook)

10 9 8 7 6 5 4 3 2 1

Contents

This book is dedicated to the River, for teaching me the joy of paddling upstream.

Everyone enjoys what is easy. The River taught me to enjoy what is hard.

Squint

Foreword

by Matt Paxton
Downsizing Expert and Host of *Legacy List
with Matt Paxton* and *HOARDERS*

"What on earth is she going to do next?"
Those were the words that many of us who know
Margit Novack said when we heard she was retiring.
I'm lucky enough to truly know Margit—an I-look-
forward-to-getting-a-random-phone-call-from-her kind
of knowing a person. She introduced me to the world of
Senior Move Management more than a decade ago by
literally grabbing my arm, walking me through a trade-
show hall and introducing me to anyone and everyone
I needed to meet. I was a kid, scared to death, entering
a room where I knew no one and every single person I
met was a strong, powerful and successful woman that
Margit had inspired, encouraged or taught as they started
their own businesses. I still remember how confident she
was as she walked me through the room and made every
single person stop what they were doing to meet me.

I've since gone on to know Margit as a mentor, a colleague, later as a business partner and now as a life-long friend. As cheesy as it sounds, this lady wears a lot of hats. She is half mom, half teacher and all warrior. For many successful women, it's difficult to find the right combination of warrior and mom. Let me assure you, Margit knows the right mix and that spirit guides you through the chapters of this book as she—and all of us readers—are educated by her interactions with clients.

This book is a great look back through her career in helping seniors downsize and move toward new beginnings. We quickly find out that Margit did much more than moving, she helped create the industry that had a front-row seat to modern aging. How lucky are we as readers to experience the best of her stories from dynamic and fascinating clients along the way. As a life-long teacher, Margit Novack uses *Squint: Re-visioning the Second Half of Life* as a tool to teach us to listen, truly listen. This book doesn't have all the answers, but the stories and experiences will guide you to a better understanding of what you'll do in your next chapter.

I hear Margit's voice as I read these stories. It's made me think back on my life, my grandparents, and all the people who helped me to become the person I am today. I have a feeling you'll see and hear your loved ones throughout these pages as you laugh and, most likely, cry a little. It's an enjoyable read that will leave you contemplating her words long after you've put the book down. My hope for you is that *Squint: Re-visioning the Second Half of Life* will do for you exactly what Margit did for me so many years ago. I hope her stories and advice grab you by the arm and walk you through your next phase with confidence. Regardless of age, grab a pen and paper and be ready to start thinking about your next act.

—Matt Paxton

Introduction

⌒⌒⌒

"We don't see things as they are,
we see them as we are."
–ATTRIBUTED TO ANAÏS NIN

Squinting is a well-established strategy that helps artists improve and transform their art. Squinting helps the artist re-evaluate their work and form a second opinion. Sometimes squinting is used to bring subjects into sharper focus, sometimes to simplify and better see the whole. In what is called the "multiple squint," several works are placed side by side and viewed as a group. Artists use the multiple squint to enhance contrast and gain a better understanding of their stylistic direction.[1]

As I look back over my personal and professional life, squinting has been a useful tool for me as well. Some edges blur, others come into sharper focus. Experiences placed side-by-side show me how I've evolved and sometimes surprise me by their juxtaposition. Above all, I see everything with a new perspective.

It's not that events have changed; it's that I'm now seeing them through the lens of a seventy-year-old. In so many ways, I'm seeing things anew, and what an interesting learning experience it's been.

I'm a Leading Edge Baby Boomer, which means I was born between 1946 and 1955 and came of age during the Vietnam era. There are about 38 million of us. We were raised with traditional values and expectations but encountered a world on the brink of tremendous social change. Many of us got college and graduate degrees. We married, had children, and moved up the corporate ladder.

Once in a while, if you're very lucky, you have an opportunity to devote your energy, passion, and skills to something you ardently believe in. In my mid-forties, I left the corporate world and pivoted to become an entrepreneur. In 1996, I founded Moving Solutions, a business to help older adults and their families deal with the emotional and physical obstacles of downsizing and moving. Friends and family wished me luck, while they probably wondered who would buy such a service. No matter—it was the right business at the right time. We filled a need in services to seniors, and, supported by senior living trends and demographics, we thrived.

I was in the business of aging as much as I was in the business of moving. I learned about gerontology so I could better serve clients and became active in organizations that supported senior issues. Recognizing the importance of what we were doing, in 1999, the American Society on Aging[2] named Moving Solutions Business of the Year. National media told our story. We were featured in the *New York Times*, the *Wall Street Journal*, the *Washington*

Post, the *San Francisco Chronicle*, the *Dallas Morning News*, *Forbes Magazine*, the *Kiplinger* report, *Time* magazine, and more.[3]

Seeing the opportunity, people from around the country sought me out for help in starting businesses like Moving Solutions. In 2002, I brought together the handful of similar companies from across the country and we gave birth to the National Association of Senior Move Managers (www.nasmm.org).[4] Invigorated by fellow entrepreneurs who shared our vision and values, we developed a code of ethics and training materials. I became NASMM's founding president and chaired its ethics committee. We were on the ground floor of a new industry. It was exhilarating.

For the next twenty-five years, I managed Moving Solutions and led and was inspired by an amazing team of individuals who shared my commitment to making a difference in people's lives.

Along the way I somehow aged and began navigating life's second half. Kids grew up, moved out, and moved back; family members became old, and I became a caregiver. Intellectually, I knew that one day I would need to envision life after Moving Solutions. In 2018, my business was acquired by a national firm, and in 2020, I set out to explore my next chapter.

I've always loved stories and the craft of writing, so my purpose seemed clear. I would write about my life and about twenty-five years with Moving Solutions. I would write about aging and the senior living industry, about relationships, about the impact of possessions and the challenge of parting with them, and about my own experience moving from middle age to young old age.

I would use stories, because stories are memorable, and because they help us connect to our emotions and to one another. I would write about what I had lived and what I had learned. I had a plan.

As I looked back, however, I realized that my stories were also part of bigger stories that were shared by others. This didn't diminish the uniqueness of my experiences. Rather, it caused me to revisit my past, this time with deeper understanding, acceptance, and appreciation. When we realize that our stories are part of bigger stories, we don't lose our uniqueness—we connect with our humanity. My stories, along with these bigger stories, became the framework for this book.

The purpose of this book is to create a positive perspective about getting older: not to sugarcoat reality, but to combat pervasive negative stereotypes about aging and to share the potential for growth and possibility. Aging includes significant challenges, but there are remarkable opportunities as well.

———•———

The second half of life includes loss; yet it is not all about loss. I have seen extraordinary grit, grace, and resilience. I have seen people explore new passions, find meaningful new relationships, give back, and create purpose. I have seen people declare their ninth and tenth decades to be the happiest years of their lives.

———•———

As described by David Solie in his book *How to Say It to Seniors*, one of the primary tasks of older adults is to examine their lives. With the enhanced perspective of age, they search for the legacy by which they'll be remembered and reflect on what their lives have meant— to themselves, their loved ones, and the world at large.[5]

As Solie suggests, I am reexamining my life. I am moving forward by looking backward. Using squints to see more clearly, I find that life is expansive with opportunity.

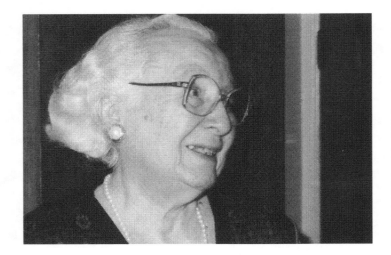

PART 1

The Bubbie Chronicles

⸙⸜⸝⸞

My husband, Bill, grew up above a small family-owned restaurant that his parents operated for three decades in Atlantic City, New Jersey. It was located next to Convention Hall during the Atlantic City heyday. Occasionally, celebrities like Dean Martin, Frank Sinatra, and Jerry Lewis would visit the restaurant for a milkshake.

One person who came in frequently for breakfast was BobbyAnn, who wore eye makeup and men's clothing. Bill remembers BobbyAnn as quiet, polite, and a good tipper, but the ten-year-old was confused. "Is BobbyAnn a man or a woman?" Bill asked his mother.

"BobbyAnn is our friend," his mother replied. With a few simple words, my mother-in-law taught acceptance and tolerance.

Bubbie was my mother-in-law, my friend, my advisor, and my muse. She was a wise woman and a great listener, patient and attentive, with a genuine interest in people. Part One describes Bubbie's journey during the last fifteen years of her life, and our journey with her.

I

Tough Love

Tough love is a concept normally applied to the actions of parents toward children, not children toward parents. But perhaps this norm needs to change. As children, we are taught to honor our parents, but does honoring your parents require that you acquiesce to their wishes? How do you balance love and respect with risk and responsibility?

My future husband took me to meet his parents. The next day, my birthday, his father died. To this day, my husband celebrates my birthday with a yahrzeit (memorial) candle.

After her husband died, my mother-in-law moved in with her daughter, Laura, and her son-in-law, Paul. The living situation started out well. Bubbie was engaged and engaging, enjoyed Laura and Paul's friends, and welcomed outings and new experiences. Then, gradually, things changed.

Bubbie became anxious; we don't know why. She asked her doctor for Valium to help with her anxiety, and thus began Bubbie's multi-year journey with Valium. Valium is prescribed to treat anxiety, pain, insomnia and panic attacks, but can also cause paranoid and suicidal ideation, impaired memory, poor judgment, and loss of coordination. [1]

Soon Bubbie developed an aversion to going out. She became suspicious and critical of Paul. Increasingly anxious, she asked her doctor for more Valium. The situation grew tense. When Laura and Paul decided to move from New Jersey to Florida, we were not surprised that Bubbie chose not to move with them. Instead, she decided to live with us.

Bill and I had reservations. We both worked full time; no one would be with Bubbie during the day. The reason we didn't want to say out loud was that Bubbie was hard to live with. Everything was too much for her. She declined to have meals with us because we ate too early or too late. She refused to go out, was critical and withdrawn, and opted often to be by herself, either sleeping or watching TV.

We felt she would be better off in a senior living residence, where there would be people to talk to. Reluctantly, she agreed to visit several. She disliked them all, but disliked one less than the others. So she moved to the Charles C. Knox Home, where she had a private bedroom and shared common space with eighteen other residents. [2] She remained unhappy.

We arranged an appointment with a social worker who did home visits; she cancelled it. "You're depressed," we told her. "I'm not depressed," she said. "I'm anxious, and my doctor agrees with me."

Anxiety and depression are both among the most common mental health disorders in the United States. Neither is a symptom of the other, but they share many of the same symptoms so diagnosis can be challenging. Doctors are less likely to recognize depression in older adults than they are in younger people, in part because medical conditions common among the elderly can cause depressive symptoms, as can medications used to treat those conditions. Some doctors attribute signs of depression and anxiety to normal aging, but depression and anxiety are not part of normal aging. [3]

Soon everything made Bubbie anxious, and Valium became her method of choice to get through the day. When we argued that her use of Valium was excessive, she countered with, "My doctor prescribes it." That was a compelling argument, since her physician was well regarded in the community and had a large geriatric practice.

We contacted her doctor and shared our concerns. "She's set in her ways and will not change," he responded. "Besides, the pills are only 2 milligrams."

"But she takes them all day long," we said. He seemed disinterested.

•———————•

It's hard to say when dependence on a medication becomes an addiction, when an aversion to going outside becomes a phobia, when a person moves from set in her ways to obstinate and rigid.

•———————•

Looking back, none of us recalled a particular date. We remembered instead a period of time over which a person we loved and enjoyed became increasingly inflexible, bitter, and withdrawn. When, we wondered, did we begin accepting this diminished version of Bubbie? When did we let go of the woman we had known and allow this stranger to take her place?

A construction project brought the situation to a head. Since Bubbie spent so much time in her bedroom at the Knox Home, we offered to build a small sitting room adjacent to her bedroom, add a private bathroom, and create a small suite. The suite would give her the privacy she lacked, since the shared bathroom bothered her greatly. In spite of this, Bubbie wanted none of it. "My life is awful and having an apartment won't make it better. Besides, dust and noise from the construction will make me ill."

Bubbie didn't want change, but she was also bitterly unhappy with the status quo. We had a window of opportunity. If we didn't move ahead, the empty bedroom next to Bubbie would be rented and creating the suite would no longer be an option. We persevered and did what we thought would be best for her; despite Bubbie's discomfort, construction began. We are not sure why, but within days, Bubbie's prediction became true. Her blood pressure skyrocketed and she was hospitalized. The next day, she called with a request: "Bring me 30 Valium, a pad of paper, and the phone number of Dr. Kevorkian."[4] Alarmed especially at her request to contact the "suicide doctor," we called her physician. "She is talking about suicide," we told him. "We want her off Valium."

"She'll never accept going off Valium," he insisted. He was right. She didn't accept it. We did it anyway. Benzodiazepines like Valium have been established as highly addictive and have significant risk factors for falls in the elderly, but stopping them is uncomfortable for both doctor and patient. We certainly saw this with Bubbie and her doctor. Perhaps this is why many doctors continue prescribing them.[5]

That evening, my husband fired Bubbie's doctor and hired another one. The new physician agreed that Valium was a depressant and that Bubbie was abusing it. She felt Bubbie would do better if she were off Valium and on a geriatric dosage of an antidepressant like Zoloft.

"She will be in the hospital for several more days, and while she is here, we can control what medications she takes," the new doctor said. "If you want her off Valium, this is your window to make that happen." She warned us that detoxing from Valium would not be pleasant, and that Bubbie would be very angry.

We didn't use the term "intervention" at the time, but that's what we did. It was a hard decision to make, and even harder to carry out. Over the next week, while Bubbie was weaned off Valium and put on Zoloft, she was furious. "I'm a mentally competent adult, and you're treating me like a child," she fumed. "You're forcing me to accept an apartment I don't want and taking away Valium—the one thing that's helped my anxiety. Why can't you leave me alone?"

Bill spent every day in the hospital with his mother, from morning 'til night. She yelled at him and cursed the day he was born. In order to do what he believed was right, my husband caused his mother pain and incurred her wrath. To this day, I am astonished at his strength, courage, and endurance.

The days immediately after Bubbie's discharge from the hospital were scary. She seemed subdued, but disoriented. Bubbie had been miserable, true, but she hadn't been confused or disoriented. What had we done? we wondered.

Soon, however, her confusion lifted. What emerged was a new Bubbie, not simply the pre-Valium Bubbie— rather, a new, improved version who proceeded to astonish us with her wit, wisdom, and joy.

The next ten years were what Bubbie described as the best years of her life. She played computer card games, read three or four books each week, and received hundreds of emails from friends and family. She knitted sweaters for both living and yet-to-be-conceived great-grandchildren.("I may not be alive when they're born, and why shouldn't they have sweaters too?") She was interested in everyone and was a terrific listener. They were the best years of our life with her, as well. Bubbie was a source of inspiration and guidance whose wisdom, wit, and warmth made her a beacon for all around her.

Ironically, Bubbie seemed to remember little about her Valium-addicted days. "I wasn't very happy then, was I?" she asked. We're glad that her memory of that time was hazy. Her new self was so much more . . . well, the real Bubbie.

When she got off Valium, Bubbie began a geriatric dosage of Zoloft, which she continued until her death.

Although she had occasional periods of anxiety, she never asked her new doctor for Valium. She told us that she had a wonderful life and felt fortunate to be alive.

Bill and I often think back to that horrendous week when, against her wishes, we had Bubbie taken off Valium. We wonder what would have happened if we hadn't been willing to use tough love with Bubbie.

Helping someone you care about when they don't want help is complex. What do you do if you believe your parents are unsafe or, worse yet, harming themselves? When do you honor their wishes, and when do you impose your own conviction that you are correct? This is an issue adult children increasingly face as their parents age. We faced this question with Bubbie. It was among the hardest things we've ever done, but also one of the most important.

2

Medication Management

 ⌒‿⌒

Like many older adults, Bubbie took a lot of different medications. On top of twelve prescriptions and
three types of eye drops, she took two stool softeners and
three vitamins. Some pills were taken once daily, some
twice, some before meals, some with meals, and some
before bedtime, for a total of nineteen pills each day.

Bubbie was mentally competent and able to manage
her medications and prescription renewals. She understood her conditions and the importance of medication
compliance, so she was careful to take each medication
exactly as directed on the bottle. She managed her medications just fine—except it seemed more and more that
her medications managed her.

One prescription bottle, scheduled for noon, said:
"Take on an empty stomach."

Another pill due at noon said: "Take after lunch."

A medication to be taken with breakfast called for
two additional dosages six hours apart. Since breakfast at

her senior residence was served at 8 a.m., she took these pills at 8 a.m., 2 p.m. and 8 p.m.

A medication to be taken three times daily said: "Take every eight hours." Her doctor told her to take this "when you wake up." Since she woke at 7, she took these pills at 7 a.m., 3 p.m. and 11 p.m. She went to sleep around 9 p.m., so she set her alarm for 11 p.m. each night to get up and take her last pill.

In order to be a good, compliant patient, Bubbie was taking pills at 7 a.m., 8 a.m., noon (before lunch) and noon (after lunch), 2 p.m., 3 p.m., 5 p.m. (before dinner), and 5 p.m. (after dinner), 9 p.m. and 11 p.m. When we commented that she was being a bit too rigid with her schedule, Bubbie showed us the instructions on the prescription bottles. She wanted to be a good patient and was adamant that the schedule had to be followed to the letter. We suggested she discuss her medication schedule with her physician, but Bubbie would never dream of questioning her doctor. So, the medication regimen continued. Constantly worried about her next dosage, Bubbie's medication schedule became an impediment to going out and doing things. ("I have to be home to take my medicine!") Plus, taking medicine so often made Bubbie see herself as sickly.

It's common for older adults to have "prescription cascade," where side effects of one drug are interpreted as a new condition, resulting in a new medication being prescribed.[1] Other than stool softeners to address a side effect of her medications, Bubbie did not have prescription cascade.

Many older adults have fragmented care because they see multiple specialists who are unaware of prescriptions given by other physicians.[2] Bubbie's care was managed by a primary care doctor who was aware of all her medications. She was taking the right medications, managed by a knowledgeable and competent physician, who followed timing and dosage instructions on the package insert. The doctor took into consideration Bubbie's height, weight, age, sex, chronic conditions, other medications, and medication intolerance . . . all the right things, except one: how the medication schedule impacted Bubbie's daily life.

When a urinary tract infection led to Bubbie being hospitalized, my husband and I spoke with her physician. We showed the doctor what Bubbie's daily routine looked like and how the medication schedule impacted her quality of life. "Isn't there some way this can be improved?" we asked.

To our delight, the doctor organized the nineteen pills into four groups instead of the previous ten. "What about the instructions on the prescription bottles?" we asked. The doctor assured us that the adjustments she made would not reduce the medications' effectiveness. She made notes in Bubbie's chart to revise instructions on future renewals. Although initially hesitant, Bubbie agreed to the revised, doctor-approved medication schedule. We found a weekly pill organizer with four sections per day, and Bubbie agreed to give it a try.

Bubbie continued to manage her medication administration. I took over prescription renewals, filled the weekly pill organizers, and soon built up a month's supply of each drug so there were no more emergency trips to the pharmacy. The new system made our lives easier, and we hoped would improve Bubbie's life as well. It did. Bubbie was happy to have the burden of renewals lifted off her shoulders. But there were other changes as well. With just four administrations daily and the pills already sorted, Bubbie began seeing herself as less sickly and started going out more. Her world became larger. Bubbie continued to manage her medications carefully, but her medications no longer managed her.

Bubbie's seeing herself as healthier was important. Studies show that people with positive perceptions of their health live longer and are healthier than those with negative perceptions.[3]

When Bubbie saw herself as less sick, she became more active. This in turn enabled her to have more experiences and a richer, more fulfilling life. All of this was made possible by a small change in routine.

Never underestimate the impact of a small change.

3

Technology Adoption

Although many older adults are intimidated by technology and push back when family members try to introduce it, those who embrace technology often find new passions. The trick is finding a way to create the first encounter. We strategized how to introduce Bubbie to email, and we succeeded beyond our wildest expectations.

Since Bubbie was an avid card player, we thought she would enjoy computer card games, but she resisted. Like many people of her generation, Bubbie did not go to college. She dropped out after eighth grade to help support her younger brother and sister. Computers and keyboards intimidated her.

We developed a plan. Bubbie often helped me assemble handouts for my business. We usually worked at our kitchen table, but this time I suggested we use my office.

I placed the material on a workstation and brought up solitaire on the computer. As Bubbie sat down and prepared to work, she pointed to the monitor and asked, "What's that?"

"It's a card game," I replied. "Don't worry about it. Let's just collate the papers."

Ten minutes later, "How do I move the jack onto the queen?" she asked. I showed her how to work the mouse. That was the end of collating for the day.

By the following week, we had installed a computer in Bubbie's sitting room and she was spending several hours per day on solitaire. We offered to show her other card games, but she said solitaire was enough. She had solitaire and the telephone; she was fine.

And for a while, she *was* fine. Then her hearing deteriorated. Loss of hearing is common as people age, affecting approximately one-third of adults 65-74, and nearly half of those over 75.[1] Like most people, Bubbie was able to compensate, but using the telephone became increasingly difficult. The high-pitched voices of her great-grandchildren were especially hard to hear.

Helen Keller is quoted as saying, "Blindness separates us from things, but deafness separates us from people." Hearing loss was eroding Bubbie's ability to connect with others. We worried that as using the telephone got harder, her world would get smaller, and she would be lonely. We took Bubbie for a hearing aid consultation, but when she heard the price, she refused to consider them. (By the time Bubbie agreed to get hearing aids—two years later—she had lost all hearing in one ear and only needed one hearing aid, which reduced the cost by 50 percent. Bubbie was pleased that by delaying she had saved so much money.)

Since Bubbie already used a computer for solitaire, we suggested she try email, where her hearing loss wouldn't be a problem. She refused this as well. Bubbie was stubborn, but so were we. We learned about a combination email printer/mail service that enabled someone to receive email without a computer. We opened an account for Bubbie and registered friends and family so they could send emails. The printer only accepted emails from registered users, so Bubbie would never receive spam. It was a perfect solution!

We set up the printer, and Bubbie announced, "I don't want it. If people send emails, no one will call me."

"They will call you," we assured her.

The printer used a regular phone line, like a fax machine, so the phone rang when an email was received. "How will I know if I should answer the phone?" Bubbie asked.

"We'll program the printer to print the emails once daily, while you're at dinner, so you won't have to worry whether to pick up the phone when it rings," we responded. She still wasn't convinced.

Since the printer was already here and hooked up, we struck a deal: We told her that if she didn't like it by the end of the week, we'd give it away.

Bubbie went down to dinner. When she returned, a dozen emails had printed out. Her great-grandchildren had scanned in their homework and two art projects. Her daughter had sent humor and health tips. Cousins sent newsy email letters. Family friends sent political commentary. An army of people had been mobilized to make Bubbie's first email experience glorious, and it was. We heard all about it when Bubbie called the next day with an urgent problem.

"Bill, the machine says it has a paper jam," said Bubbie.

"Okay, Mom," said Bill. "I'll be over tomorrow morning to fix it."

"Tomorrow morning? What happens to emails that arrive tonight?"

One day of email, and Bubbie was hooked.

Bubbie's email interests were eclectic. She liked letters, news, and health information. She liked political commentary, puzzles, and humor. She loved art and school projects from her great-grandchildren. Soon dinners were cut short. "I have to get back to my room," she'd say. "I have mail."

Within a few weeks, Bubbie learned how to refill paper and clear paper jams on her own.

"How come you never send me email?" she asked Bill one day.

"Mom, we're right here. We see you every day. Why would we send you email?" said Bill.

"Everyone else does," she replied.

In her ninth decade, Bubbie had learned something new and conquered something that had intimidated her. Being part of the "high-tech world" made her feel young. Plus, email gave her stories to tell and information to share. Bubbie loved to communicate.

Physically, Bubbie's world was small: a bedroom, bathroom, and modest sitting room. But emotionally, Bubbie's world was large. She had meaningful relationships, was passionate about world events, and conquered

In her ninth decade, Bubbie had learned something new and conquered something that had intimidated her. new challenges. Bubbie's large world was made possible by many things—caring friends and family, an understanding physician, a special bird (more about that later), and by email. As Bubbie's hearing continued to deteriorate, email helped her stay connected with friends and family.

Hearing loss is not a cognitive impairment, but scientists have found that people who have hearing loss are more likely to develop dementia than people without hearing loss. Hearing loss also leads to social disengagement, isolation, and depression, all of which may accelerate cognitive decline.[2] *Technology did more than bring Bubbie joy and help her remain connected and engaged— it may have helped her thrive cognitively as well.*

4

Difficult Conversations

It is important to have honest discussions with loved ones about how they want to spend their last days and what they want for their funeral. According to Ellen Goodman, co-founder of The Conversation Project, the difference between a "good" death and a difficult death is whether someone has shared how they want to live at the end of life and die. Surveys show that 90 percent of people think it's important to have this conversation, yet only 30 percent of us have actually had it. Family members often hesitate to initiate the discussion; they worry it will offend their loved one or that it feels too early. "The truth is that it always feels too early, until it's too late," says Goodman.[1] Sometimes a daughter-in-law can have conversations that are too hard for a son or daughter. I had "the conversation" with Bubbie. It flowed naturally and wasn't awkward. Bubbie and I were both glad we did it.

The conversation started when I told Bubbie that I had attended a networking meeting held in a funeral home. I described how the funeral director talked about personalized funerals, where people defined exactly what they wanted for their funeral.

"I want to do that," said Bubbie, "It's my funeral. I want to be in control."

And so we began. I learned that Bubbie did not want hymns; she wanted "Stardust Memories," a favorite song she'd shared with her husband, Herm. Except for her wedding ring, she did not want to be buried with jewelry. "Dead is dead," she said. "Let someone else use it."

I asked if she wanted to be buried with any books (Bubbie loved to read). She considered Conroy's *The Prince of Tides* but decided against it. "Perhaps a crossword puzzle and a pen," she said. "I don't plan to erase." For the funeral meal, she wanted nothing low-salt. "I've had to watch salt for the past thirty years. No Alpine Lace at my funeral." When asked what clothing she wanted to be buried in, she said, "My pink sweatsuit and sneakers."

"A sweatsuit and sneakers?" I asked.

"Yes," she replied. "I am not wearing pantyhose for eternity."

Next, we talked about caskets. Bubbie wanted the least expensive that could be found. "I am pretty short," she said. "Do you think I could fit in one of your wardrobe cartons? I would be dust-to-dust really fast. It would be very green."

I burst out laughing. Bubbie was clearly enjoying herself. This conversation led to other conversations, which included her advance directive and end-of-life preferences. And so it was, when Bubbie died several years later, that there were no questions about what she wanted. She died in her sleep, on her recliner, with a crossword puzzle on her lap, so there was no need to refer to her advance directive. As for her funeral, she had it her way.

●────────●

Articles about having "the conversation" stress how difficult it is to initiate end-of-life discussions. What they don't discuss enough is how satisfying these discussions can be for the older adult.

Bubbie had strong opinions we wouldn't have known or guessed. Talking about her end-of-life wishes made her feel in control. Looking back, I am so grateful to have had this conversation with Bubbie. It was a gift we gave one another.

Additional resources for initiating end-of-life conversations can be found in the chapter notes at the end of the book.[2]

5

The Importance
of Being Needed

The period of life after a person reaches sixty-five is sometimes referred to as the "third age," a time characterized by disengagement from paid and socially valued roles. While this leads to enhanced well-being for some people, it contributes to lack of purpose for others. Older adults don't lose their desire to be valued and useful; these feelings are crucial to physical and mental well-being. Studies show that older adults who feel needed are less likely to die or require institutionalized care. For older adults in particular, purpose matters.[1]

When my husband was growing up, his family had a series of songbirds, canaries, and parakeets, each named Pookie—so it seemed only natural that the green and yellow parakeet we acquired would be dubbed Pookie as well.

Pookie didn't strike me as a very exciting pet. He didn't sing. He didn't talk. He didn't do much of anything. That is, except when Bubbie would visit. Having nurtured the entire Pookie dynasty, Bubbie knew ways of talking to birds that were foreign to me. Her voice assumed a certain inflection, she gave Pookie her undivided attention, and five minutes later, he was singing and chirping away.

"Why don't you take Pookie?" we asked.

"I don't want a bird," she replied. "Too much trouble, too much responsibility. No way."

One day, our cat made a leap for Pookie's cage. Although the bird was uninjured, its near-fatal adventure inspired us, and we developed a plan. We would be visiting friends, we told Bubbie. Could she keep Pookie overnight until we returned and could rehang the cage?

Bubbie sensed a plot, but reluctantly agreed. "Okay," she said, "but pick him up the second you get home." We delivered Pookie to her apartment. She was so busy talking to him she didn't notice when we left.

When we called the next morning to schedule Pookie's pickup, she said, "Let's negotiate. Pookie stays here."

So began the friendship of Pookie and Bubbie. Certainly, the relationship was good for Pookie. He played with toys, chirped and sang constantly, and occasionally even talked. But it was clear that Pookie gave more than he received. According to my mother-in-law, he was "the smartest bird that ever lived." He made her laugh. He provided company. He was a friend and, perhaps most important, Pookie needed her.

Like many people of her generation, my mother-in-law had had a hard life. She began working as a young girl while caring for her brothers and sisters. As a married woman, she and her husband operated a small restaurant and lived above it in a tiny apartment where they raised their family (and multiple generations of Pookies). A good listener, Bubbie was sought after by friends and family for her counsel. She played a vital role in many lives.

At eighty-five, however, my mother-in-law was a widow who no longer worked. Her children and grandchildren were grown and self-sufficient. Few people depended on her for nurturing or advice; instead, she depended on others. Pookie made a difference in her life. Each morning, she got up to change Pookie's water, replenish his food, adjust his toys, and, of course, talk to him. Twice monthly, she went to Petco to buy supplies, and she cleaned Pookie's cage. In short, Pookie depended on Bubbie.

Bubbie recognized Pookie's importance. "I depend on folks at the Knox Home for food and housecleaning. I depend on you and Bill for trips to doctors, for shopping, and for my medications, but Pookie depends on me. It feels good to be needed."

Then, Bubbie fell and broke her hip. At first, she was reluctant to begin physical rehab. When we told Bubbie that some people never return to independent living after a hip fracture, she said, "Give me the walker. I have to get better so I can go home and take care of Pookie."

In the meantime, we needed someone to care for Pookie until Bubbie's discharge. Our daughter bravely volunteered. Two days later, she called. "How's Pookie?"

we asked. "Not good," she said. "He is lying at the bottom of the cage with his feet in the air." There was a collective groan as we shared the news with family members near and far. Caring for Pookie was Bubbie's reason to get well. Not only would Pookie's death make her sad, we were certain she would refuse to get another bird.

I am the first to admit that I am not a bird person. To me, a bird is a bird. But I am a person of action. I took the still-warm Pookie in his crate and headed to our local Petco. The manager saw me with a dead bird and assumed I was there to complain. "You don't understand," I said. I explained the whole saga and how we needed a bird that looked just like Pookie.

We searched the parakeet area, which housed dozens of birds, but none of them looked remotely like Pookie. "How much time do we have before she gets out of rehab?" asked the manager. I happily noticed he said "we."

"About a month," I said.

"I have seven stores in my region," he told me. "I'll check every one for a parakeet that looks like Pookie." Using his cell phone to capture Pookie's likeness, he gave me his phone number and email address. I left the store astonished, grateful, and committed to shopping at Petco for the rest of my life.

The entire family was in on the hoax. My daughter, who cannot tell a lie, stopped visiting Bubbie, lest she burst out crying. My son, who lies easily, started setting the stage. He told Bubbie that he had visited Pookie, that Pookie really missed her and was pining away. "In fact," he said, "Pookie looks like a different bird."

I called the manager two weeks later. He had been to four stores with no luck. "Don't worry," he reassured me. "I still have three stores to go." Meanwhile, Bubbie was making steady progress.

A month after entering rehab, with no advance warning, we were informed that Bubbie would be discharged the next day. Panicked, I called Petco and asked for the manager. "He's on vacation for two weeks," said the person on the phone.

"Oh no," I groaned. "He was getting me a bird."

"Wait, are you looking for Pookie Novack?" the clerk asked.

"Yes!"

I rushed to the store. In the back was a very thin, very quiet, but definitely Pookie-ish parakeet. "Thank you, God," I said, and the new Pookie and I went home.

The next day, Bubbie returned to her apartment. Leaning on her walker, she walked slowly into the room and settled into her recliner. She looked at her small sitting room, her family pictures, and her bird. "Pookie," she said, "I am so glad to see you." Phew, we had passed the first test!

We called the next day. "How is Pookie?" we asked.

"He's a little thin," she replied. "He must have been traumatized by my being away. But he's coming around. He hasn't stopped singing."

As the months passed, it became clear we had pulled off the switch of the century. We were grateful to everyone who helped in our conspiracy of love, but especially to the manager at Petco, who understood the power of pets in the lives of older adults and the importance of being needed.

My mother-in-law read the *New York Times Book Review*, did crossword puzzles, and was addicted to solitaire. Not too much got past her. "Do you think she doesn't know it's a different bird?" friends asked. "She must know and not be telling you."

"If she does know, she doesn't care," Bill and I replied. "She is busy loving the bird she has."

"It's the weirdest thing," Bubbie said a few months later. "Pookie plays with toys he never played with before." No doubt about it: Pookie was one happy bird.

After Bubbie passed away, we found Pookie a new home, but he died soon after. We like to think it's because he missed Bubbie so much and couldn't wait to join her. We never did find out if Bubbie knew about the switch, but it doesn't matter. We are thankful that Bubbie spent her last years loving her bird and feeling needed.

Bubbie didn't replace my mom, but she filled a hole in my heart. Her sense of humor, her fierce intelligence, and her ability to truly listen and not judge, drew me and others to her. She was a blessing in my life, and every time I think of her, I smile.

PART 2
Revising My
Personal Narrative

One of the most important developmental tasks as we age is to review important relationships and events in our lives. As I looked back, I had many "aha" moments, in part because my perspective had changed. But the most disconcerting aspect of reviewing my past was how imperfect my memory of it is. For example, my mother came to the US from Hungary when she was twelve. She had a strong accent, which everyone but me seems to remember.

My recollections of the past form much of how I see myself. If I could misremember something as obvious as my mother's accent, what else about my past could I be misremembering?

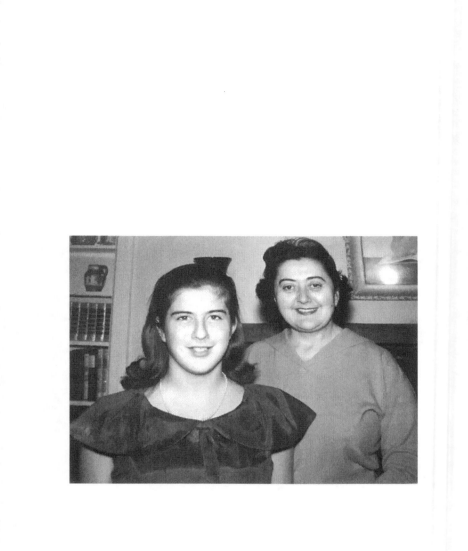

6

Mother-Daughter

If you're a midlife orphan, your parents were alive for most of your adult life. You danced with your father at your wedding; you shared joy with your mother when your children were born. You were able to show your parents the person you became, and your children were able to know their grandparents. As your parents grew older, you were able to return the nurturing and love they gave you.

That's why I am confused by many midlife orphans. They complain about caregiving responsibilities, and then when their parents pass away, they lament being orphans. They are bereft, unmoored, devastated by life without parents. Don't they realize how lucky they are? Yes, they should mourn their parents' loss, but they should be glad for the time they had with them, too. Navigating the caregiving of elderly parents is complicated, often challenging. But having elderly parents is a privilege some of us never had.

I became an orphan when I was young. My dad died when I was seven; my mom, when I was twenty-six.

I was devastated when I learned my mother's cancer was terminal. For months, I grieved for the life events we would never share: my wedding, the birth of my children, the grown-up me she would never know. To this day, I have daydreams of conversations with her. "Look Mom," I say. "Don't worry about me. I'm okay. I have a wonderful husband and three grown children. I started a business and helped launch an industry. I have a great life. Are you proud of me?"

I guess we never stop wanting our parents to be proud of us.

I have many memories of my mom, but the one that stands out most is the last time I was mothered. It didn't seem special at the time. My mother had been in the hospital for nine months. Today, the infusions she received would be given as an outpatient procedure, but this was 1976. It was my twenty-sixth birthday, and my boyfriend had done nothing, not even given me a card. I walked into my mother's hospital room. "Hi, honey. Happy birthday," she said. I burst out crying and told her why I was so upset. My mother held me, and I was comforted.

It wasn't until years later that I recognized the gift I had received and, perhaps also, the gift I had given. For months, I had been managing my mother's affairs, dealing with doctors, paying medical bills, being the grown-up. I so longed to feel like a child again, and that night, my mom gave me that gift.

For months, my mom had been the sick one, the patient. As a single mom who had raised three children on her own, how unfamiliar it must have been for her to be so dependent on others. I realize now what I couldn't see when I was younger—how much she needed to feel like a mother again. That was the gift I gave her that evening.

•————————•

Most of all, I remember how exquisite it felt to be mothered. Here I am, forty-four years later, myself a mother and grandmother, and I still yearn for that feeling.

•————————•

So perhaps I do get it, why midlife orphans are so devastated when their parents die. No matter our age, our parents are such a primal connection that their loss leaves us missing a part of who we are. One thing is certain: I will always remember the last time I was mothered. I will never be loved like that again.

The play Our Town, *by Thornton Wilder, was a popular school performance when I was growing up. Although I have forgotten much of it, I remember snippets, especially when Emily Webb returns from the dead on her twelfth birthday to see her family once more. Her happiness turns to pain as she realizes how little people appreciate the simple joys of life. Every moment of life, she realizes, should be treasured. I understand. I would treasure being with my mom for even one moment.*

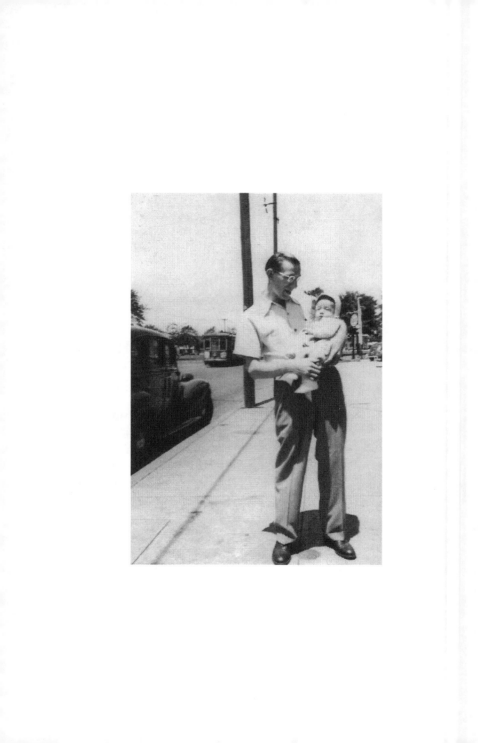

7

Father-Daughter

I was only seven when my dad died, so I don't remember much of what it was like to have a father. But I remember what it was like not to have one. I grew up in the fifties, when almost no one was divorced. As a child, I didn't know anyone who didn't have two parents—just my brothers and me.

When I was eight or nine, our synagogue held a father-daughter event. In order for me to attend, a member of the Men's Club offered to serve as a stand-in father. It was a kind gesture, but I remember thinking how ridiculous it was. Nothing makes a fatherless girl feel worse than a stranger serving as a stand-in father.

I remember having daydreams as a kid, that my father was away doing some kind of clandestine research for the government (this was during the Cold War) and that he would one day reappear in my life. The reappearance was always during an assembly program, where my astonishment was seen by all—the kind of dramatic reveal you see on reality TV shows. I never dwelt on why the government wanted a near-sighted pharmacist for research.

I do have one especially fond memory of my dad. It was the first warm day in spring. I must have been in first grade. I came running into my parents' bedroom (by this time my father was bedridden with the bad heart he would soon die of) and asked my dad for help getting into a pair of shorts. I had grown a great deal since the summer, and there was no way those shorts would fit, but I was determined. "Push me into them, Daddy!" I remember saying. "Make them fit."

Nothing could make them fit. Laughing, he called my mom and said, "You'd better bring home some larger shorts."

I'm not embarrassed by my determination at age seven. It was such an accurate predictor of the drive and stubbornness that have defined me my whole life. They are at once my best and worst qualities. I am glad that my dad saw this part of me and loved me in spite of it.

Throughout my life, I never felt I missed anything by not having a father. That is why I was so surprised when, several years ago, I had such a strong reaction to simple gestures I saw between two fathers and their daughters. In one instance, a father twirled his daughter's hair. In the other instance, a daughter played with her father's fingers. These two mindless acts of intimacy created such a longing in me to have had a father, to have been somebody's little girl, it was visceral. I was shocked. How could I, who hadn't thought about my father in decades, yearn so much for what I hardly even knew? Just as I started to process the feeling, it was gone. I felt cheated. I wanted it back. I wanted to experience what it felt like to miss my father.

I wish I knew more about my dad. I wish I had more memories of him. But perhaps, in my recollection of the shorts that did not fit, I already have the most important memory. I remember being so imperfect and still being loved.

Maybe that is the gift we get from our parents. They see all of us, our best and worst qualities, and love us in spite of them.

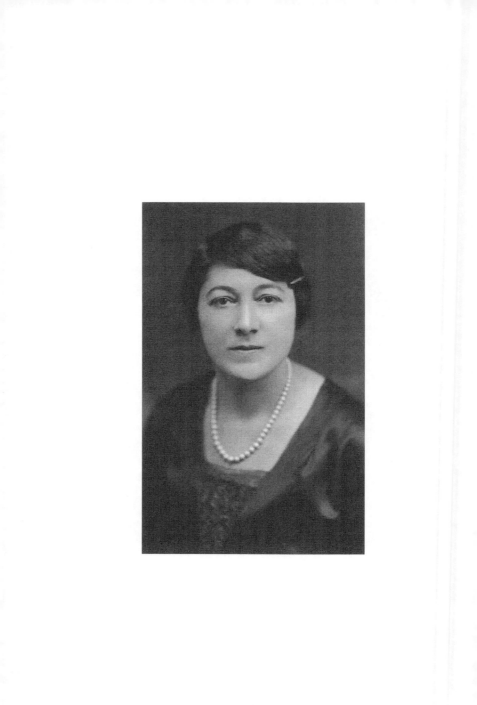

8

Detaching with Love

How do you care for a family member who is critical, impossible to please, or emotionally abusive? Many mental health professionals suggest "detaching with love." Although detaching with love is traditionally applied when one person is struggling with addiction, it can be used in contentious relationships too. You affirm your love for the person but also make it clear that you will not tolerate their behavior. Detaching with love does not judge someone, control their actions, or imply approval; it means setting clear boundaries and allowing the person to deal with the consequences of their decisions. The need to detach with love transcends any one particular age bracket.[1]

My grandmother was a hoot. She was also relentlessly critical—not of other people, just of me. To stop her constant criticism, I had to detach with love. But it is so much more complicated than that.

Everyone called my grandmother Anya, the Hungarian word for mother. She became a widow with two children when she was twenty-one. In 1931, without knowing any English, Anya left her children with her parents in Hungary and came to America to make a better life for herself and her family. Two years later, she married a widower and brought my mother and uncle to this country.

Life during the Great Depression was hard for Anya (and for millions of others), but, over time, she lived the American dream. She started businesses, and, although many of them failed, some succeeded. Her son became a doctor, and her daughter married a pharmacist. Both had single family homes in the suburbs.

From my earliest memories, Anya ran guest houses in Atlantic City and headed bazaars for the Hebrew Old Age Home. She was a strong woman, a force to be reckoned with. I remember that she and my mom argued frequently when I was a child. Although they spoke in Hungarian, there was always a sprinkling of English, so I understood that the arguments were often about how my mom was raising me and my brothers.

After my mom died, Anya transferred her opinion-sharing to me. I could say she was a product of her time, that mothers are harder on daughters and granddaughters than they are on sons and grandsons. We all have thoughts we choose not to share, because sharing them would be hurtful to others. However, Anya did not hesitate to share her opinions of me.

"Anya, I got my hair cut."

"Really? Most people try to look better after a haircut."

And: "Margit, why is there a number on the back of your T-shirt?"

"It's from a work-sponsored baseball team I'm part of."

"Oh, I thought you were a prisoner."

Many of her comments centered around her fear that I would never get married.

"Anya, I'm getting a master's degree."

"A master's degree? Who cares about a master's if you're not a missus?"

And: "Anya, this is my new cat."

"No man will marry a woman with two cats."

"How can you say that?"

"Are you married?"

"No man will marry a woman who walks barefoot..."

"No man will marry a woman who eats raw cookie dough..."

"No man will marry a woman with a sofa."

In my early thirties, I accomplished what she'd feared would never happen. I got engaged.

"Anya, I met a wonderful man, and we're engaged. He is Jewish, has a Ph.D., and is divorced."

"A divorced man? A divorced man is like a squeezed lemon. No juice left."

Now that I was getting married, Anya had more to say—lots more.

"How can you marry a man who left his wife and children?"

"He didn't leave his children, they are with us all the time."

"Oy vey, all the time."

"Anya, I went shopping for an antique wedding dress."

"A used dress? Might as well, you have a used husband."

Our wedding invitations were not traditional, but they were the invitations we wanted. A calligrapher created the design, we had the invitations printed, and the children and I hand-colored them with magic markers. It was a group project—the perfect invitation for our new family. Immediately, we got a call from Anya.

"Do you children need money?"

"Why Anya?"

"Because I just received the invitation and it is cheap. You will get cheap gifts. I will give you money so you can get real invitations, with tissue in between."

"Anya, we chose these invitations. We like them."

"Why do you like cheap invitations?"

Finally, the big day arrived. We had a lovely wedding in the horticultural center, with high-top tables and food stations of contemporary cuisine. I went to Anya during the reception, kissed her, and asked, "Anya, are you happy?"

"How can I be happy?" she said. "The food's not fit for pigs."

This was harsh, but she could not ruin my day.

The next morning, she called and asked for the name of the caterer.

"Why?"

"So I can report him to the Better Business Bureau."

That did it. I had had enough. I did what I had never done before, perhaps what I should have done earlier.

"Anya, it is NOT OKAY for you to criticize my wedding. You would never go to someone's home for dinner and complain to your hosts about what they served. You cannot criticize the food at my wedding."

"I am telling you the truth because I love you."

"That is not love."

Then she played her trump card: "Don't worry, I'll be dead soon."

At this point, I was crying, she was crying, but I didn't back down. "Anya, I don't want you to be dead. I love you. But I want you to hear this and to hear it clearly. You cannot continue to criticize my husband or my wedding. If you say one more negative thing about either, I will stop visiting you."

More tears from both of us, and I hung up.

I don't believe Anya changed her opinion about my husband or the wedding, but I know she heard me. While she continued to share opinions on many topics, she never criticized Bill or my wedding again.

Looking back, what I feel most sad about is not her comments, it's that she wouldn't share my joy. She had no living children. I had no parents. We both had voids to fill. My marriage should have been a time of happiness, of healing. Anya didn't ruin my happiness, but together we both could have had more.

Should I have said something to Anya sooner? For years, I had dismissed her comments, telling myself, "She buried three husbands, two children, and one grandchild.

She is entitled to be difficult." When those close to me said, "You should tell her to stop," I would reply, "It's Anya, she'll never change." I had more control than I realized, but I never exercised it.

Maybe there is no such thing as "should have done it sooner." Perhaps we all have to arrive at our personal last straw before we detach with love. That is how I arrived at mine.

●————————●

Detaching with love is hard, especially when it concerns a parent or grandparent who we naturally want to please and respect. However, the cost of not setting boundaries is high.

●————————●

Keeping my grandmother at arm's length emotionally helped me tolerate her comments but prevented us from having a close relationship. She became a caricature instead of a person. By not detaching with love sooner, we both lost.

As I was writing this book, I spoke about this story with my brother. "I always respected how you kept your promise to Mom that you wouldn't fight with Anya," he said.

"What promise?" I asked.

"The one you made to Mom in the hospital, the night before she died."

I did feel I was honoring my mom by not arguing with Anya, but I have absolutely no recollection of a deathbed promise made to my mother, or even a discussion with her about Anya. How can I have forgotten such an important conversation? Maybe my subconscious remembered it, and that is what motivated me to keep quiet for so long. I will never know.

9

Senior Suicide

People sixty-five and older make up 12 percent of the population but account for 18 percent of suicides. This percentage increases as people get older and is highest for those over age eighty-five. Experts believe that senior suicide is likely underreported by 40 percent or more, since "silent suicides," like deaths from overdoses, self-starvation, and dehydration, are often not included. Young people have a higher incidence of attempted suicides, but older adults have a higher rate of completed suicides. [1]

Studies cite major depression, misuse of alcohol, and psychiatric illness as contributing factors to senior suicide, which paints those who attempt or commit suicide as mentally ill or "broken." For older adults who face loss of independence, financial problems, grief, and unrelenting pain, depression may be a rational response to a future of unacceptable options, and suicide a desperate attempt to retain control.

Thirty years ago, Anya, at ninety-two, tried to kill herself. They called us from her personal care residence to say she had been found unresponsive with an empty bottle of pills by her bed. My brother Mark and I rushed to the hospital and listened to her stomach being pumped. For anyone who has never heard it before, it's an awful sound. My brother and I looked at each other and wondered, what if they hadn't found her in time? Shouldn't a ninety-two-year-old be able to say when enough is enough?[2]

All of Anya's relatives, including her sister and her parents, had been killed in concentration camps. Pain from persistent shingles, pleurisy, and arthritis was constant. When doctors gave her enough medicine to control her pain, she was too lethargic to live independently. So she faced her own brand of Sophie's Choice—live with pain and be independent, or have controlled pain but live in a nursing home. Anya opted for a third choice.

When we saw her the next morning, Anya was disoriented and did not mention her failed suicide attempt. While hospitalized, she met with a psychiatrist who told us she was depressed. "She has good reason to be depressed," we said. "She's had loss after loss, and now she's about to lose her independence." The next day, Anya was discharged to a nursing home where she shared a room with three other women. Two weeks later, we received a message on our answering machine that she had died.

I had mixed feelings. Anya was the last tie to my mother. Letting go of that bond was hard. Yet I knew what independence had meant to Anya. I understood her decision. Faced with no good options, Anya found a third choice. It was the right choice for her.

For years, when my husband wanted to annoy me, he would say, "You're just like Anya." I knew he was referring to her stubbornness and domineering personality, so I took it as the insult he intended. But over time, I've come to realize that I probably am a lot like Anya. Like Anya, I am determined, driven, a force to be reckoned with. Why is that a bad thing? A lot of good things get accomplished by people who are driven and determined. I am proud of being a force to be reckoned with. That is why, twenty years later, when my children asked what my grandchildren should call me, I told them, "Call me Anya."

Logic suggests that grieving for a parent or grandparent with whom you had a strained relationship should be less intense than when the relationship is close. Experts think the opposite is true. When there is unfinished business, you aren't able to resolve your issues. Many people find this unbearable. Losing someone with whom you had a challenging relationship, they explain, adds a new layer of grief: loss of the relationship that might have been.[3] This resonates with me.

Articles about grandparents suggest the relationship between grandparents and grandchildren is based on love, appreciation, and pure joy, that there is a special bond. I didn't have that with Anya. I don't grieve loss of my grandmother as much as loss of the relationship we could have had.

Losing someone with whom you had a challenging relationship, adds a new layer of grief: loss of the relationship that might have been.

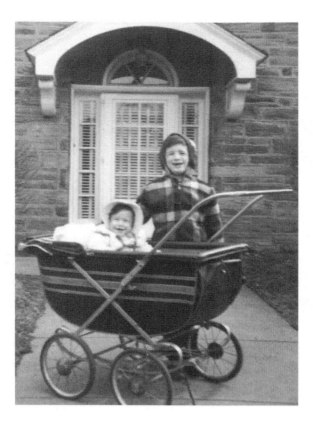

10

Sibling Estrangement

Sibling estrangement is a hidden but surprisingly common phenomenon. It's estimated 5 percent of people with siblings are estranged from a brother or sister, and this figure is likely under-reported. Experts believe that sibling estrangements are on the rise. Major life changes such as marriage, divorce, birth, illness, or death can trigger a separation between siblings, but this usually only occurs if tensions have been building for years.

"Sometimes, estranged siblings are struck by a sudden yearning to reconnect . . . but breaking the ice is hard," writes Lise Funderberg in her article in *Time* magazine, "Why We Break Up with Our Siblings."[1] I was one of the 5 percent of adults who are estranged from a sibling. Several years ago, I reached out. I'm glad I did.

I hadn't spoken to my oldest brother, Michael, for many years. Like most cases of family estrangement, the ostensible cause wasn't the real cause; we'd had a bad relationship for years. So, it's not surprising that when our mom died, we argued over what would happen to her things. There were things I wanted (all of which I got) and things I didn't want for myself but didn't want Michael to have. I told myself it was because he wouldn't take care of my mom's things. Looking back, I'm not sure why I had that conviction.

One particular argument was over my mom's blue sofa. We had words, and then we had more words. Then X happened at my wedding, and Y happened two years later, and soon, we had no relationship. Occasional, rare phone calls reinforced my position that I didn't feel or want a bond with him, and soon decades passed.

A few years ago, a friend told me the story of two former prisoners. Both had suffered horribly in confinement. One prisoner told the other he had forgiven his captors. The other said he could never do that. "Then you are still a prisoner," the first prisoner replied.

I hadn't thought about Michael in years. Yet, just like that, in an instant, I decided to end the estrangement. It wasn't a question of forgiveness. I had spent forty years of my life angry at my brother. It was time to move on.

And so I visited him. During that visit I learned many things. Michael was quirky and sometimes tactless, but he was not the ogre I had imagined all these years. The blue sofa I was sure he wouldn't take care of was still in his living room, well-loved and covered with my mom's crocheted afghan. I would not have kept a fifty-year-old blue velvet French Provincial sofa, I realized. I would have gotten rid of it. Although very different in our approaches, we had both been good stewards of our mother's treasures.

This past year, I came across letters I exchanged with Michael forty-plus years ago. As I read them, I ached at my young arrogance and harsh judgments. Clearly, I had misremembered some things, and over the next four decades these misremembered memories became part of a personal narrative that supported our estrangement.

I wouldn't say that my brother and I are now reconciled. Letting go of hostility does not reinstate a close relationship. We are very different people, and there is a lot of history that can't be erased. But I no longer feel anger, and have in its place sadness and, perhaps, humility. I am less certain of things than I used to be and more aware that some of the memories that define my past are flawed. Ending estrangement, it turns out, only requires accepting that what we believed, what we thought was so, may not be the way it really was. That is a beginning, and perhaps a beginning is enough.

When I called Michael and asked if I could visit, we never talked about the past. We simply moved on. Neither of us was interested in assigning blame. Clearly, we are both different from our younger selves. According to experts, the ability to overlook imperfections for the sake of relationship is a hallmark of maturity. At seventy-five and seventy, it appears that Michael and I are at last mature.

I'm glad I reached out to Michael, but reaching out is not a guarantee of success. According to Terry Hargrave, family therapist and author of Families and Forgiveness, about 40 percent of families who attempt reconciliation fail, mostly because no one is willing to take responsibility for what happened.[2] Perhaps there is another way to succeed at reconciliation: instead of looking back, simply move forward.

> According to experts, the ability to overlook imperfections for the sake of relationship is a hallmark of maturity.

II

Personal Treasures

As a Senior Move Manager, I saw firsthand how difficult it can be to part with items inherited from family members. And not just heirlooms; even ordinary items can carry with them a sense of responsibility. These items represent a family's legacy. Letting go of them feels like betrayal, disrespect, or lack of appropriate stewardship.

I felt this way about parting with items from my family as well, until I realized I was safeguarding the wrong thing. When my mom died, I got many of her things, and among my favorites was a glass cake plate. It wasn't fancy—not etched or cut glass. It had simple, elegant lines, and I had always liked it. My mom and I used to bake together, and this had been her favorite cake plate, so after she died, it became my go-to cake plate as well.

One day, I made a cake for a friend's party, and, as usual, used my mom's cake plate. At the end of the party, half the cake was left over, so I left the cake plate and told my friend I would get it later.

The next day, I received a call from my friend. "Please tell me this cake plate wasn't a family heirloom."

"It belonged to my mom, who died, and it's one of my favorite things," I replied.

Dead silence.

Then I said, "But my mom is in my heart and my mind . . . not in a cake plate."

What was I supposed to say? It was clear the cake plate was kaput. But what I had said was true. My mom didn't live in material things; she lived in my memory. I thought about my children, who never knew my mom, and then I realized something else, something more.

My mom came to this country when she was twelve, and she was put back a year in school to learn English. When she was sixteen, she contracted tuberculosis and spent a year in a sanitarium. When she got out, she was two years behind in school. She never finished high school. This was an important part of my childhood. From the time I was small, I knew that my mom's lack of education bothered her. Sometimes when she met the parents of my friends, she would say, "I didn't go to college, but I think I am just as smart as they are."

She was so smart, and she loved to read. Whatever I was reading in school she would read too, and we talked about the books. Together, we read Willa Cather, *My Antonia* and Richard Llewellyn, *How Green Was My Valley*. I read *Le Petit Prince* in French; she read it in English. We read Calderón and García Lorca. How we loved discussing literature!

My mom was more than smart; she was resilient and wise. Widowed at thirty-eight, she raised three children alone. When I was offered free room and board at college, my mom said, "I think you should live in the dorm."

"I thought I was going to commute," I said. "You want me to live away?"

"I didn't raise you to stay at home," she said.

The thing is, if I want my children to know their grandmother, they won't learn about her from a cake plate. They will come to know her from stories that I share. I was being a good steward of my mother's possessions—what she owned—but not of who she was. Who she was is communicated through stories, and if the stories are passed down, the possessions become immaterial.

It's not just inherited items that have stories. Sometimes items we gather through our lives acquire stories, and that's when they become personal treasures. If you visited my home, you wouldn't notice my personal treasures, even though they're in plain view. They have no material value, but they have special meaning to me.

One treasure is a blue and white mug, a souvenir from a trip to the Bahamas with my friend Karen when we were both single. For years, the mug had no special meaning. I kept it on my desk to hold pens. Eight years after our trip, Karen, at age thirty-six, was diagnosed with advanced breast cancer and died. During this same time period, I was diagnosed with breast cancer too—except that, thirty-two years later, I am alive and well. Why was I so fortunate, and Karen so unlucky? Life seems so arbitrary; it's hard to make sense of it. That's why, over time, that ordinary blue mug has taken on new importance. It reminds me that life is unpredictable and that I should not take things for granted. That's a message worth passing on.

One of my favorite stories is from a friend. When my friend was growing up, one of her mother's most prized possessions was a large brass bowl. Her mom polished the bowl regularly and gave it a place of prominence on the sideboard in their dining room. One day, my friend brought a boy home to meet her parents, and her mother served dinner in the dining room. Her boyfriend was nervous, and it's possible the liver her mother served didn't help matters. Whatever the cause, during dinner the boy became obviously ill, and just as he was about to throw up my friend grabbed the closest thing she could find for him to throw up in—the brass bowl.

Fast-forward forty years: the boy who threw up became her husband, and her now-elderly mother had passed away. As she and her sister went through her mom's apartment, she asked, "Where's Mom's brass bowl?"

"She gave it to me years ago," her sister replied. "She was afraid it would embarrass you because of what happened at that first dinner."

"Are you kidding?" my friend replied. "That bowl has been part of family stories for decades. We tell it again and again. The brass bowl is a personal treasure to us *because* of what happened." All those years, my friend hadn't owned the bowl, but that never diminished her joy in telling the story. The story, not the bowl, was the treasure. That's the thing about personal treasures.

Like the velveteen rabbit who becomes real over time, personal treasures don't start out as treasures; they evolve, and even when the item no longer exists, the story continues to bring happiness.

> We all have items inherited from family members, and these become a special kind of burden when we try to downsize. "How can I part with my dad's tool chest, my grandmother's china?"

Like the velveteen rabbit who becomes real over time, personal treasures don't start out as treasures; they evolve, and even when the item no longer exists, the story continues to bring happiness.

In his book Downsizing: Confronting Our Possessions in Later Life, *Professor David Eckert writes about "safe passage," the process of leaving things that belonged to people we loved to those who we think will value, appreciate, and care for them.[1]*

I wonder if we are providing safe passage for the wrong things. The people we loved are in our hearts and our minds, not in what they owned. We honor them by safeguarding and passing on their memory. It's stories, not possessions, that need safe passage.

12

Blended Families

From time to time, when something doesn't go my way, I find myself saying, "What am I, the red-headed stepchild?"

The term "red-headed stepchild" describes a person who is neglected, mistreated, or unwanted.[1] The phrase has its origins in America in the early 1900s. It's a horrible, anachronistic phrase, and it's all the more surprising that I use it because being a stepmother is one of the best things that ever happened to me.

Two of my three children were born before I met them. They were five and eight years old when I married their dad. They are good, decent people. I would love to take partial credit, but they achieved this on their own. On the other hand, they have definitely helped me become a better person. While being any kind of mom teaches you many lessons, being a stepmom teaches additional lessons, including one that impacts me to this day.

It all started with socks and underwear. I would send the kids to their mom's wearing new socks and underwear, and they would return wearing old ones. Oh, how it annoyed me! I would tell the kids to wear the new socks and underwear back to our house, embroiling them in an ongoing battle over something insignificant. Finally, I got it. It's just socks and underwear. I bought a larger supply and stopped worrying about which ones came home.

Decades passed before I truly assimilated the lesson I was given. I continued to grumble about this or that until one day, I saw the similarity to my struggle with the socks and underwear. Now, when I lose perspective about something unimportant, I say to myself, "It's like socks and underwear," and let it go. What a gift I received!

Over the years, I have received many gifts from my children, both the one I gave birth to and the two that I met after they were born. Together, I believe we avoided many of the complex issues blended families can go through. Perhaps we were lucky, but maybe it wasn't luck. Perhaps we all stepped up to the plate to make our relationship succeed.

Today, it's adult stepchildren who are stepping up as they care for aging parents and stepparents, and I hope my stepchildren will do this for me when the time comes. But my stepchildren have known me since they were young; we've been together for thirty-eight years. For many stepchildren, this isn't the case. They are caring for stepparents they acquired as adults when their parents entered into late-life marriages.

Caring for aging parents is challenging when you share the burden with siblings you grew up with, let alone stepsiblings you met as adults. It's easy to fall into an adult version of socks and underwear: "I do more for my stepmom than her own children do." Eventually we realize that keeping score is pointless because everyone loses, so we let it go. Stepchildren who are great caregivers don't step up because of a scorecard. They step up because of who they are.

Caring for aging parents is challenging when you share the burden with siblings you grew up with, let alone stepsiblings you met as adults. It's easy to fall into an adult version of socks and underwear.

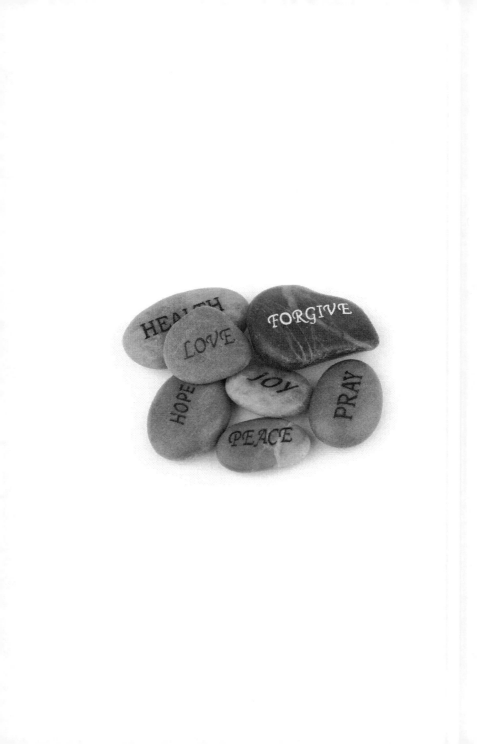

13

Forgiveness

My husband and I collect stones with words on them: love, health, family, even *beshert* (a Yiddish word meaning soulmate). We had thought our collection was complete, but realized one was missing, so we added a new stone: forgive.

Forgiveness is a central theme of the Jewish High Holidays. We ask God to forgive our sins, and we forgive those who have wronged us. What I don't see emphasized is the need to forgive ourselves. Self-forgiveness, the ability to say, "Who I was before doesn't dictate who I will be in the future," seems to be at the core of atonement.

I often think about a sentence I heard at a WW (Weight Watchers) meeting. Your eating can be out of control at 10:00 and back in control at 10:05.

I love the insight this phrase suggests. It speaks to the hopeful premise that whatever your failings, you can forgive yourself, change, and move on. Forgiving yourself, however, is harder than you might think.

I can list many things I've done as a parent that I'm proud of, but I have a wall of shame as well. When my children were young, I was a yeller. Every parent yells at their kids at times, but I yelled a lot. One day, when my daughter was twelve, we went to the grocery store. I gave her a list of things to get. When we met at the check-out counter, she had gotten one wrong item, and I yelled at her. A few minutes later, a woman approached me in the parking lot and said, "You don't know me, but I saw you shout at your daughter in the grocery store. Do you even hear yourself?" I started crying, not from embarrassment that I had been reprimanded by a stranger, but because I knew she was right. I yelled too easily and too often.

Later that afternoon, I told my daughter how sorry I was and promised to try to yell less in the future. I was unsure how successful I'd be; I knew how entrenched my behavior was.

I didn't expect or deserve my daughter's response. "It's been a really hard year," she said. "You've had breast cancer, and Dad has a lung condition. I know you don't mean to yell as much as you do. You've been under a lot of stress." Here I was, the mom, being comforted by my daughter. She forgave me, but I did not.

I remember a conversation I had with my mom when I was in my early twenties. She confided that my older brother, Michael, had wanted to go to Hebrew high school, but she had discouraged it because she hoped he would go out for football. "Can you imagine?" she said. "He barely did anything that required sneakers, and I thought he would want to play football. He had no father, so I thought he needed to be around sports. What a stupid, stupid decision."

At some point you realize that your parents are human. They made the best decisions they could at the time. My brother might have forgiven my mom, but she hadn't forgiven herself.

I smile when I hear young parents agonize over how long a time out should be or when to remove a pacifier. "Relax," I want to say. "There will be things you'll do right and things you'll wish you had done differently. Just do the best you can." Thankfully, our kids tend to forgive us. I am not sure when we forgive ourselves.

That's why the Weight Watchers message is so important. It is a reminder that our future doesn't have to be dictated by our past. Whatever our regrets about the past, tomorrow we can do better. Who knew Weight Watchers had so much to say about atonement?

Self-forgiveness is important for people of all ages, but especially for older adults. Studies suggest that self-unforgiveness is directly related to poor mental health, including depression, rumination, negativity, pessimism, and hopelessness.

•————————•

Reflecting on the past is an opportunity to do internal housekeeping, to let go of negative thought processes that diminish joy and satisfaction in the present, and to move forward.[1, 2]

•————————•

What an adventure I have had reviewing my personal narrative. I was, at turns, comforted, enriched, surprised, troubled, and humbled. I learned that my memory is imperfect and my perspective, evolving; that perception is malleable, and the past is always shifting. When I changed the way I looked at things, the things I looked at changed.

Looking back was so, so worthwhile.

PART 3

Becoming

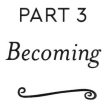

I feel vibrant and alive, but there is no denying that my body is changing. It's not that I'm aging; I prefer to say that I'm *becoming*.

Becoming, as a verb, suggests evolving into a new state. As an adjective, it means attractive, enhancing, flattering. Perfect—I'm becoming!

Becoming suggests "process," a journey more than a destination, which seems appropriate. As I look back, I can see that I'm still myself, but I'm also evolving.

Take hats, for example. I have never worn hats—not in winter, not in summer. I'm categorically not a hat person. Yet this year I began wearing hats in cold weather. I now marvel at how exquisite it feels to have a warm, comfortable head.

I am changing in other ways, too. When I worked in the corporate world, I treated myself to special jewelry every year. These days, what I used to spend on jewelry I now spend on yoga and Pilates. Instead of focusing on how I look, I'm focusing on how I feel.

Instead of focusing on how I look, I'm focusing on how I feel.

By the time we reach a certain age, we think we know who we are and what we like, and that these attributes are static. It turns out they're more fluid than we imagined. These days, I see priorities as something malleable, like butter or Jell-O—things that change shape under different circumstances.

I now love things I thought I hated. I no longer care for things I thought I loved. What else might I like if I were open to change? Am I hanging on to ideas about who I am or what I must have, even if these ideas no longer serve me? Are these ideas preventing me from evolving, keeping me from new experiences that might enrich my life? These are questions I ponder.

14

Letting Go of Ageism

As life spans grow longer, the definition of "old" is changing. According to Sergei Scherbov, lead researcher of a multi-year study on aging, "Someone who is sixty years old today is middle-aged." [1]

When does old begin? Scherbov says for Americans, it's roughly seventy to seventy-one for men, and seventy-three to seventy-four for women, but your true age is not just the number of years you've lived. The idea of his study is that the threshold for old age should not be fixed but depend instead on characteristics such as life expectancy, personal health, cognitive function, and disability.

Of course, the meaning of "old" also depends on who you ask. Young people think fifty or sixty is the onset of old. People in their forties say the onset of old is sixty-five. Folks sixty and older say it's about fifteen years older than their current age. According to Scherbov, I am not old yet— although at seventy, I am definitely getting old-ish.

A wintry mix was coming down outside, and as I put on my boots I thought, I don't want to fall.

"You sound old," I said to myself.

And then I thought, Why does not wanting to fall make me sound old? I think it makes me sound smart.

With its bold portrayal of female sexuality, Erica Jong's 1973 novel, *Fear of Flying*, resonated with women my age. We were part of the women's movement; we were creating social change!

When did fear of flying become fear of falling?

I started to think about risk-taking. Risk-taking is highest in adolescents and tends to decrease as we age. Is that because older adults are more fearful or because they're more experienced? Being cautious and prudent should make me wise, so why did I see it as "being old?"

Am I ageist?

The term "ageism" was coined in 1969 by physician/gerontologist Robert Neil Butler, who was the first director of the National Institute on Aging. Butler defined "ageism" as:

1) Prejudicial attitudes toward older people, old age, and the aging process;
2) Discriminatory practices toward older people;
3) Institutional practices and policies that perpetuate negative stereotypes about older adults.[2]

In his book *Healthy Aging*, Dr. Andrew Weil asked people to list attributes associated with "old."[3] The words frequently cited included ancient, antiquated, dated, dried up, frail, passé, shriveled, used up, useless, withered, worthless, and wrinkled.

Why aren't wise, accomplished, experienced, mature, and capable associated with "old?" Ageism is so commonplace in today's society that we don't even recognize the stereotypes implicit in many things we say and feel. We grow up believing and perpetuating these stereotypes even as we become older ourselves.

All of this sounds theoretical, but in fact it's quite personal. Studies show that older adults who equate aging with becoming useless, helpless, and devalued are less likely to seek preventive medical care, are more likely to suffer memory loss and poor physical functioning, and die earlier.

When aging is seen as something positive, however, the opposite is true. Older adults who view aging as a time of wisdom, self-realization, and satisfaction live seven and a half years longer than those with negative views. That is a bigger benefit than not smoking![4]

So what does this mean for me? If I want to thrive as I age, it's not just external ageism I need to watch out for; it's internal ageism as well. I need to be

> Being cautious and prudent should make me wise, so why did I see it as "being old?"

mindful of my own negative views about getting older. My boots are a good start. Being cautious about falling is not being old; it's being wise.

Despite my good intentions, fighting internal ageism is hard. I saw a cute dress recently, an inch or two above the knee, with chic black and white stripes, and it flowed nicely when I moved . . . I wanted it. I stood in

Older adults who view aging as a time of wisdom, self-realization, and satisfaction live seven and a half years longer than those with negative views. That is a bigger benefit than not smoking!

line at the checkout counter, and then I thought, Am I too old to wear this?

While younger women sometimes ask this question, it's especially prevalent among older women. We ask this question because we don't want to be judged as inappropriate by others, and we know this happens because *we* judge others. We look at other women and think to ourselves, They're too old to wear that. We've appointed ourselves the clothing police for others, and in doing so, we end up policing ourselves.

The Internet is filled with articles on what styles you can wear at thirty, forty, and fifty. Some articles reach as high as sixty, but after that, apparently, your choices are limited. You can be current, but not too current, with everything worn "in moderation." The articles warn women not to use clothing to try to "look young." They're missing the point. Clothing isn't just about how you look; it's also about how you feel. What's wrong with wearing clothes that make you feel good? At this point in our lives, we should dress to please ourselves, be more comfortable stepping outside our comfort zone, and be less concerned with what others think. With considerable enthusiasm, I made a manifesto.

When I am old, I shall wear purple and . . . cropped pants, and leggings, shoes with ankle straps, camisoles, large purses, black nail polish, and more. I shall wear things that are comfortable and that make me happy. I won't worry that I will be judged by others, and I will try not to judge others as well.

Then I walked into a restaurant, saw a woman ten years older than me in an off-the-shoulder top, and thought, She's too old to wear that.

So much for my manifesto. Letting go of ageism is a work in progress. I'm evolving, and I have much work to do.

A few years ago, I was at an Apple Store, asking a question about my iPad, when the twenty-something young man helping me said, "I really like the way you highlight your hair."

I stared at him, dumbfounded.

"Really," he said, "the way the blond blends in with the gray is very attractive."

I thought to myself, Is this some new sales technique? If so, it's working. I'll take an iMac, a MacBook Air, an iWatch, an iPad, and three iPhones.

As I left the store smiling, I thought about how pleasant it was to receive a compliment about my appearance. After a certain age, women don't expect to receive compliments about their appearance, especially from young men. We become accustomed to being invisible. Society doesn't see old features as being beautiful—but I do.

I've thought about times I've complimented older women, even simple statements like, "You have beautiful eyes." Their whole face lights up, because receiving a compliment about their appearance is such an infrequent occurrence. What an easy way to give a moment of happiness, and it makes me happy, too. I resolve to do this more often. In the meantime, there is still something wrong with my iPad. I may need to go back to the Apple store.

15

Why My Purse
Was in the Freezer

I've studied the aging process for twenty-five years. As we get older, short-term memory loss increases and brain processing speed slows down. This is referred to as normal, age-related memory loss. Some people experience more than normal age-related memory loss. This is referred to as mild cognitive impairment (or MCI). People with normal age-related memory loss and people with MCI can live independent, meaningful lives.

Five million people in the US, and 50 percent of people above age eighty-five, have some degree of dementia. Dementia includes memory loss, but is also characterized by problems with judgment, language, and abstract thinking and interferes with daily and social functioning.[1]

Memory lapses can be frustrating, but they are not the same as dementia, and most of the time they aren't cause for concern. I know this, but sometimes it's hard not to wonder what's normal and what's not.

A few weeks ago, I found my purse in the freezer. After appropriate jokes about a new meaning for the term "cold cash," I considered what this might actually mean. Did finding my purse in the freezer mean that I had mild cognitive impairment or early dementia? I began doing what many people above a certain age do when they forget something or notice cognitive changes: I worried if finding my purse in the freezer was a sign of something serious.

I began a self-check.

Was I forgetting things like people's names, where I placed my keys, or where I parked? Yes, but I have always done this. Although aggravating, this is common for me and for most people as they age. I chalked this up to normal age-related memory loss and made a silent promise to write down where I park and try to put my keys in the same location every time I come home.

Another warning sign of dementia is difficulty performing familiar tasks. I need to be retaught the rules of cribbage every time I play, but I have always been card-challenged. I didn't recall other difficulties with familiar tasks, so I crossed this symptom off my list as well.

I checked to see if I was disoriented about time and place. Was I forgetting how I got somewhere or how to get home from familiar places? I've always had a good sense of direction and still had one, so I decided I was good here as well.

Was my judgment poor or decreasing, like wearing heavy clothes on a warm day? Nothing jumped out as worrisome, so I moved on to the next symptom.

Was I having trouble with abstract thinking, like forgetting how to balance a checkbook? I used Quicken to balance my checkbook each month. I decided this was not a problem area either.

Was I putting things in unusual places, like a purse in a freezer?

Oops.

I needed to delve into this one a little further. I have a tiny purse, just big enough for my cell phone, cash and credit cards. It is black and hard to find when it's misplaced, which is often. But how did it get in the freezer?

I considered my habits. Because my purse is so small, I often place it in whatever I am carrying into the house—like a bag of bagels, for example, which is where I eventually found it when we defrosted the freezer. I decided to mull this over.

In the meantime, I ran to the store to get batteries. I reached in the bag to take out the batteries and lo and behold, there was my purse again. I concluded that given my habits, a purse in a bagel bag in the freezer, while unusual, is understandable. It wasn't a symptom of decreased judgment. It was a symptom of being distracted.

I decided that for now, I likely did not have dementia, but I am more easily distracted when I multitask. I also realized that I had crossed some age threshold after which actions that were laughed off when younger are now taken seriously. Whenever there is a mental hiccup, I now ask myself, Is this a sign of something more serious?

I am glad to have my old purse back and happy to report that six months of being frozen appears not to affect cash. (The credit cards and driver's license were replaced.) Age-related memory changes begin as early as fifty. The changes are gradual, so it may seem that there is little difference from year-to-year, but the effects are cumulative, so each year there is greater impact. At seventy, my memory has already been changing for twenty years. I feel a little different from who I was, but not much. It's part of becoming.

16

Mishearing

One of the most common problems we face as we age is hearing loss. Approximately one in three people between the ages of sixty-five and seventy-four, and nearly half of those above age seventy-five, have hearing loss. But many people don't want to admit they have trouble hearing. Fewer than one-third of people with age-related hearing loss use hearing aids. Part of the reason is cost; hearing aids are expensive and are rarely covered by insurance. But the bigger reason may be ageism. In our society, hearing loss affects how others perceive us and how we perceive ourselves. A major reason people who would benefit from hearing aids don't use them is that hearing aids mark the user as old.[1]

Consider the difference from age-related changes in eyesight, which typically begin when people are in their forties. Most people have no issue using eyeglasses or bifocals as they age, particularly with today's blended lenses. Not so with hearing loss. We typically deny it as long as we can and acknowledge it years after our spouse or partner has recognized the problem.

I've been dealing with hearing loss in my own family, but I refer to it as mishearing. "Bill, there is something wrong with the fan," I said to my husband (in another room). He walked into the kitchen, tried the cooking spray, and said, "There is nothing wrong with the PAM." Life has been interesting since we started mishearing.

A major reason people who would benefit from hearing aids don't use them is that hearing aids mark the user as old.

Sometimes we hear part of the word, but not enough to make out the actual meaning, so we fill in the void with words that make sense given the context. Our helpful brains instantly construct elaborate thought processes around what we think we heard. Often we're right, but sometimes we're not, and this creates some interesting conversations.

For example, you ask someone what he does for a living, and he responds, "I work with diabetic Jews."

Wow, you think. There's a business that works just with diabetic Jews? How are Jewish diabetics different from other diabetics? Is it something genetic? Do cultural differences make diet compliance more challenging? Of course, these thoughts all occur in nanoseconds.

"Yes," he continues. "People with diabetes often have poor circulation and need special shoes." And that's when you realize that he said diabetic *shoes*, not diabetic *Jews*.

In age-related hearing loss, the ability to distinguish between consonants is one of the first things we lose, and consonants are what help us differentiate words. We replace them with other consonants, and hence, we mishear.

Age-related hearing loss is the basis of many jokes about old people.

Three old men are out for a walk. The first says,
"It's windy today."
The second one says, "No, it's Thursday."
The third one says, "So am I. Let's go for a beer."

At first glance, these jokes are funny—but are they really? They associate hearing loss with aging and make people with hearing loss look stupid. No wonder people are reluctant to acknowledge their hearing loss.

Mishearing doesn't need to be associated with hearing loss. Consider kids reciting the Pledge of Allegiance. The kids don't have hearing loss; they just misheard and substituted words they thought made sense:

I pleger legions to the flag of the United States of
America, and tunary public, for witches hands,
one nation, on a God, invisible, with liver trees
and Justin's for all.

When kids mishear, it's cute. When older adults mishear, we see them as stupid.

Our bias about age-related hearing loss is another example of ageism, but perhaps we can change the paradigm. I was surprised, though pleased, when my husband agreed to get hearing aids after a hearing test showed he needed them. He synchs his hearing aids with his phone and iPad and listens to music and news in bed without bothering me as I read. Because of his hearing aids, not only does he hear better—we can each enjoy our preferred pastime in each other's company. Hearing aids have upsized our lives.

17

Consumer Invisibility

In theory, companies want to know how old you are so they can understand differences in priorities and spending habits. Once you reach sixty-five, however, it seems you lose the preferences that define you as an individual or part of a cohort. You become part of a group whose members presumably all think alike: the old. Forward-thinking companies are exploring service and product customization to attract and retain the sixty-five and up consumer, but mainstream companies are far behind.

I've been keeping track of surveys I receive. Many are electronic, and some are hard copies, but they all seem to have one thing in common: your opinion only counts until you reach sixty-five.

As a baby boomer, I am accustomed to feeling important, which is why I am so bothered by slowly becoming invisible. All my life, I've been courted for my influence and buying power. Once I reached sixty-five, however, my opinions weren't worth squat. In survey after survey, I am lumped into an "over sixty-five" category that assumes I think and purchase just like an eighty-five-year old, and I don't like it.

The sixty-five and over population is diverse and has significant spending power, so one would think companies would want to know a lot about us, but apparently not. I could describe this as bad marketing and leave it at that, but this practice is insidious. By lumping older adults together without age segmentation, these surveys assume that needs and values vary by life stage when you are younger, but stop varying once you are over sixty-five. Though seemingly innocuous, they're perpetuating a value system that says older adults are homogenous and don't count. They influence both younger people who take the surveys, and older adults who adopt these beliefs themselves.

I realized how institutionalized ageism is when I looked at Survey Monkey, a popular online survey creation tool. When Survey Monkey illustrates age segmentation to potential users, they use examples that say "65 or older." This leads people designing their own surveys to assume they should use "65 or older" too. Age bias that aggregates and marginalizes older adults is pervasive.

I tried being devil's advocate. Perhaps it's because many surveys are online, and they reason that people over the age of sixty-five aren't online. That's not true. According to the Pew Research Center, 67 percent of people over sixty-five use the Internet (up from 13 percent in 2000). One-third of people over seventy-five are Internet users, and one-third of people over seventy-five use smart-phones. Use of technology may not be as high in seniors as it is with younger age groups, but technology adoption by older adults is large and growing.[1]

Next, I tested another argument. Maybe individuals sixty-five and over aren't major consumers of products and services. Not so. Older adults purchase 41 percent of new cars, 25 percent of toys, and 80 percent of luxury travel.[2] You would never guess that from looking at ads, which almost always feature younger people (unless it's an ad for medication). If older adults are such significant spenders, why do businesses continue to ignore them in surveys?

I admit, for companies like Urban Outfitters and Under Armour that cater to younger populations, age segmentation beyond sixty-five may not be important. But how does that explain this Chico's customer satisfaction survey I received?

Under 25
25 – 34
35 – 44
45 – 54
55 – 64
65 or older

Based on this survey, Chico's thinks that folks under twenty-five have different opinions than those between twenty-five and thirty-four, but that people over sixty-five are so similar to those seventy-five and eighty-five, that additional age segmentation is not unnecessary. Do they think my needs and opinions as a seventy-year old, are the same as someone eighty-five? Everything about this survey perplexed me, because I've spent a lot of time in Chico's, and I've never seen anyone under thirty-five, let alone under twenty-five—but I've seen a lot of people who are sixty-five and older.

I am happy to report that some companies do see the light. Last week, I received a survey with age segmentation that went to eighty-five. I wondered what forward-thinking group realized that seniors are not all alike.

It was from a funeral home.

An AARP report on what it calls the Longevity Economy reports that Americans over fifty are taking the economy in new directions. The AARP study predicts that the economic activity to serve the needs of Americans aged fifty and older will account for more than half U.S. GDP (gross domestic product) by 2032. This includes both products and services purchased directly and further activity this spending generates. Rather than be a burden to society, says AARP, Americans fifty and older will fuel economic activity, provide employment for nearly 100 million Americans, and provide nearly 70 percent of charitable giving from individuals. I am excited by the AARP report and the changes it describes, but you wouldn't guess this is the case based on consumer surveys. [3]

18

Relationships

When someone asks my husband how long he's been married, he says, "Thirty-seven years . . . twenty-eight of the happiest years of my life." He's right, of course. Some years were way better than others.

Each marriage, like each person, is a work in progress. I sometimes wonder if I would value the highs as much as I do had I not experienced the lows. Long-term relationships reward resilience.

One fascinating aspect of resilience is how weaknesses can become strengths and vice versa. In fourth grade, they gave me a cello because I was the tallest girl in my class. In fifth grade, they took it back because I was hopelessly tone-deaf. Over the years, being tone-deaf has gotten me into a lot of trouble, but it has helped preserve important relationships as well.

For years, my husband accused me of speaking with an angry tone. This was often in seemingly innocent sentences, such as "I'll be right down." I argued that he was perceiving an angry tone where there was none.

Most of the time, I believed my argument, but sometimes I knew in my heart he was right. I don't know if I actually sounded angry, but I *was* often annoyed when he called me away from something I was in the middle of, so it's possible my voice did reflect anger. I argued that my words were neutral; he argued that my tone was not. In our house, we didn't use angry tones when we argued. Angry tones were why we argued.

I think everyone has at times wished they had a tape recorder so they could replay what was just said, to prove their innocence or someone else's guilt. The trouble is, there usually is no tape recorder playing, so we are left with our imperfect and often biased perceptions. In the middle of an argument, we seldom consider that our perception may be flawed or that our interpretation is influenced by where we are in life, in our relationship, or simply at that very moment.

I remember an incident years ago. I was ending a relationship with a boyfriend who would not commit. The final blow was when I made brownies, and he said, "These brownies are almost perfect." It was one more example of how he always held back. The next morning, I left for good. The six-month relationship was over.

As I think back to that statement, the example sounds hopelessly trivial, but it didn't seem trivial then. Arguments never do at the time. It was years before I accepted that my interpretation may have been wrong, that my dissatisfaction with the relationship may have influenced how I interpreted his sentence.

Realizing that interpretation is subjective and potentially flawed is humbling. It's also sobering, because it means that others subjectively interpret what you say as well. When it comes to interpreting things said in relationships, we are all somewhat hearing-impaired.

Yet interpreting words and tone subjectively is not always bad. My brother Mark often uses a tone with me that he seldom uses with others. Coming from anyone else, I would find it offensive, but coming from Mark, it is simply older-brother speak, and I am good with it. It is not that I don't hear the angry tone, it's that I am so certain of the love behind it that I choose not to care.

That's the good thing about being tone-deaf . . . we have a choice. We can take offense, or we can choose to ignore it and rely on our knowledge of who the person is.

It is said that 10 percent of conflicts are due to differences of opinion, and 90 percent are due to "wrong tone of voice." When I played cello, being tone-deaf was bad, but in relationships being tone-deaf can be a good thing.

Last year, on Valentine's day, someone asked me, "What valentine message would you give to your younger self?" I would send this: One day, someone will walk into your life and make you see why it never worked out with anyone else. It would have been especially helpful as I struggled through my twenties, trying to find my way in life and relationships, to know that one day I'd find someone wonderful who would love me more than I could imagine.

> It is said that 10 percent of conflicts are due to differences of opinion, and 90 percent is due to "wrong tone of voice."

I'd send this message as well: One of the hardest decisions you'll ever face in life is choosing whether to walk away or try harder, to remind myself that commitment is not always easy.

Pulling it all together, I would tell my younger self this: If you're lucky, you'll find someone terrific, someone who brings out the best in you. It won't always be easy, but lots of things that are hard are worth doing. You will always find ways to annoy one another, but in the scheme of things, they won't be important.

●————————●

Relationships are a continuum, not a point in time. Relationships are not static; they're always becoming.

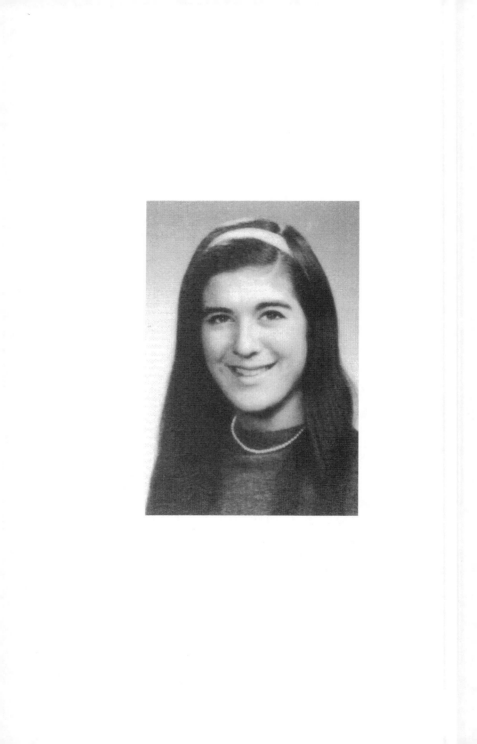

19

Diamonds in the Rough

This past year I attended a fiftieth reunion for my class at the Philadelphia High School for Girls, popularly called Girls' High. [1] I saw hundreds of accomplished, truly interesting women, women who seemed nothing like the awkward, naïve, searching girls we'd been in high school.

When diamonds are being mined, they look like volcanic rock and their surfaces are rough. Their true beauty is realized through the cutting and polishing process. This gave rise to the phrase "diamonds in the rough" to describe individuals who have hidden exceptional characteristics or potential, but who lack the "polish" that would make them stand out in the crowd.

That is what we were back in high school: diamonds in the rough. Just as diamonds are formed by years of immense pressure, we've been molded by life choices and decades of experiences. We've matured, evolved, and metamorphosed, and the brilliance of our facets has been exposed. Like diamonds, we now have depth. We are strong, beautiful, and unique.

I was a college freshman during some of the most pivotal events of the twentieth century: the Vietnam draft lottery, the 1969 moon landing, Woodstock, bastions of male-only education admitting women, the Democratic National Convention in Chicago, the first ATM, the founding of PBS, the withdrawal of troops from Vietnam, the invention of the first microprocessor.

Amidst these history-making events, I wrote about how many calories I had consumed that day, worried about course selection, ruminated over what boy I sat next to, and obsessed over my GPA. As I looked at what was important to my nineteen-year-old self, I am disappointed in my values, shocked at how mercurial I was, and struck by the fact that I didn't seem happy. Being young was way harder than I remembered.

I am happier now than I was when I was young, and it turns out I am not alone. In a study in the *Journal of Clinical Psychiatry*, researchers found that young people report the highest levels of depression, anxiety, and stress and the lowest levels of happiness, satisfaction, and well-being.

•————————•

In spite of stiffening joints, weakening muscles, fading eyesight, clouded memory, and the modern world's contempt of aging, old people are surprisingly the happiest. Across countries and cultures, research results are remarkably similar: Older adults are happier than younger people and have a greater sense of well-being.[2]

———•———

It seems that older people are better at controlling their emotions and accepting misfortune and are less prone to anger. In one study, subjects were asked to listen to recordings of people saying disparaging things about them. They found that older people were less angry than young people in the study, often taking the view, "You can't please all the people all the time." I can relate to that. Years ago, I would have been devastated if someone didn't like me. Now, I think: "Lots of people don't like me; get in line."

So, do I want to be young again? No. Like essayist and screenwriter Nora Ephron, I do feel bad about my neck, but it is what it is.[3] When bad things happen to me now, it's not the end of the world. I am resilient. I know I will live through them because I've faced challenges before. When the wind doesn't blow my way, I reset my sails.

I'll take resilience and maturity over youth any day.

PART 4

Perfection Is Not Required

Just as he began to play at Lincoln Center in New York City, violinist Itzhak Perlman broke a string on his violin. Perlman had had polio as a child and was left disabled. Getting on- and offstage with crutches is no easy task. So what did he do? He played with three strings. As the account in the *Houston Chronicle* reports, even on three strings, the performance was remarkable. When the piece ended and the thunderous applause died down, Perlman said to the audience, "You know, sometimes it is the artist's task to find out how much music you can still make with what you have left."[1]

Perhaps that is the way of life for all of us. No one expects to live life with three strings.

Yet, as we age and change physically and cognitively, for many of us, life is like living with three strings instead of four. We lose abilities but endure, we make music with what we have left. Wholeness and perfection are not required to create beauty and meaning. That is the theme of these next stories.

20

Still Someone

A client was taking me on a tour of her apartment.

"See this picture, this is me and my daughter Joan in our first house. I loved that house," she told me.

"No, Mom, that's me," her daughter Eileen corrected.

Realizing her mistake, her mother stopped and became quiet.

"Why did you have to correct her?" I thought to myself. She was telling a story. Did you see her face when you pointed out that she'd made a mistake?

I've seen this happen a hundred times—adult children correcting their parents, unable to allow an inaccurate memory even at the cost of hurting their parents' feelings. I think it's instinct, more than conscious decision, because if they thought about it, they would choose to be kind.

"**M**argie, dear, I'm moving, and I need your help." So began the call from my then ninety-one-year-old aunt Betty. Never mind that I'd been Margit for thirty-eight years. To Aunt Betty, I would always be Margie. I went to Florida to help her move from a two-bedroom apartment into a senior living community.

Betty moved to the community on a Monday, taking only two suitcases. The community provided furniture on loan until hers could be delivered. My job was to help her go through belongings at the old apartment, identify what she wanted, and have it brought to the community—in short, to help her sort through her possessions and downsize. No problem. After all, I figured, I'm a Senior Move Manager. But I was also, I discovered, a niece, and throughout the weekend these two roles collided.

Like many of my clients, Aunt Betty had a hard time parting with items I knew she would never use. Sometimes, I could cajole her into letting something go.

"But I loved this lamp," she said, pointing to a forty-inch-high lamp that was still in its shipping box from eight years earlier.

"Well, not enough to use it in the past eight years," I replied.

"You're right," she said with a laugh.

These interactions—I refer to them as reality checks—were easy because they did not diminish her as a person.

It was harder when we looked at large serving dishes.

"I may have a dinner party," she said.

Betty was frail. She used a walker and qualified for independent living only because she had aides six days per week. I couldn't say to her, "Betty, you will never have another dinner party. You haven't made a meal for yourself in months." She did not need to be reminded of this reality.

It was similar when we went through clothing she insisted she might wear someday, like a pantsuit from a dozen years earlier. I couldn't remind her that she now wore pants with elastic waists so she could pull them up herself and with seats full enough to accommodate disposable underwear. Some images of ourselves need to be preserved as who we once were, not who we are today.

Even though much of what she wanted to take would never be worn or used, I knew there was space for it in the new apartment, so I put it in the pile to go with her. Her decisions weren't always practical or wise, but they were *her* decisions, and the Senior Move Manager in me accepted that.

Later that day I met with a Move Manager colleague whose staff would handle the packing and transport of clothing and other items after I left. I took my colleague aside and said, "If you find any clothing that's torn or stained, toss it." As the words left my mouth, I was horrified. I would never say that about a client's belongings! At that moment, I realized I was no longer a Senior Move Manager: I was a family member.

The ease with which I lost professional objectivity and slid into judgment and expediency was alarming. I understand now why adult children are so often pulled in this direction. They're

> Some images of ourselves need to be preserved as who we once were, not who we are today.

coping with mixed feelings about their evolving role and added responsibilities as well as with changes they see in their aging family members. When expediency wins, it's not from lack of caring—it's from lack of energy and time.

As it turned out, the next day was when the roles of Senior Move Manager and family member were most in conflict. I had arrived Saturday morning, and Betty and I worked through the weekend. When I took her back to her new apartment, it was 8 p.m. Sunday. I dropped her at the door and suggested that she start walking toward her second-floor apartment while I unloaded my car. When I knocked on the apartment door fifteen minutes later, there was no answer. I began walking through the hallways and found Betty on the first floor.

"I got lost. I couldn't find my apartment," she said. "Then I got so tired, I had to sit down."

"Your apartment number is on your walker and also on the keys around your neck," I gently reminded her.

"I know, but I just couldn't figure it out," she said.

That's when I realized I had done it again. Like so many family members, I came in for a weekend determined to get things done in the time frame I had available. I had put my need for productivity ahead of Betty's need to rest and enjoy my visit. I wanted to be finished; Betty wanted us to have time to talk.

Betty had moved in on the previous Monday, a transition that was hard and emotional. She barely had had time to adjust when I had swooped in the following weekend and created two incredibly long and intense days. As a Senior Move Manager, I knew that stress and anxiety take an enormous toll on seniors, a toll that often manifests itself as memory loss and disorganized thinking. Whatever cognitive status Betty had before the move, the disorientation I observed Sunday night was Betty under the worst conditions. I had caused it, and I should have known better.

When I visited Betty Monday morning, I apologized for exhausting her over the weekend.

"Oh honey, I just feel so bad that you worked so hard," she said.

There she was, the Betty I knew, parenting me, rewarding me for coming down to help. Yet, in her next sentence, she was confused about whether she was in Florida or Philadelphia. The juxtaposition of the old Betty I had seen a few seconds earlier and the new, confused Betty was sobering.

In the days that followed, Betty did rebound from the stress and fatigue and began to sound more like herself. Still, she was aware she was changing. "My memory has gotten so bad," she said, clearly disturbed. "I am not the person I used to be."

To dispute what she knew to be true would be condescending. Yet I wanted her to know that even if her cognitive status was changing, to me, she was still the same person, and I still loved her.

"I have noticed a change from months ago," I responded. "I think you are about 90 percent of the Aunt Betty I know, and that's okay with me."

Betty smiled. I think being 90 percent of Aunt Betty was okay with her, too.

21

Fault Lines

One of the most difficult aspects of packing is handling items that are already damaged or that have been previously repaired. These items are especially vulnerable to repeat damage, and sometimes, no matter how careful you are, they break. Some people are especially fragile, too. Like items that have been previously repaired, the stress of moving pushes them to the breaking point.

Some time ago, we worked with a couple moving to an active adult community. They asked for help getting their home ready for listing. At our initial meeting, the wife cried, I assumed from embarrassment at the home's condition or from anxiety that we would push her to throw things away. As we later learned, the real reason was more complex.

The couple had two grown sons, both of whom lived far away. A third son had died of a drug overdose many years before and had been found in his bedroom in this house by the father. After his son's death, the father developed an alcohol problem with which he struggled ever since. As we sorted, we came upon many items that had belonged to the deceased son. It was very difficult for both parents. During the downsizing process, the husband's drinking increased, and we observed mounting tension between husband and wife. One day, we arrived at 9 a.m. to find the husband already drunk and being taken to rehab. It was not the first time, his wife informed us, and she doubted it would be the last.

"What can we do?" my staff asked. "How can we help them?"

"We can do what they have hired us to do in a caring and professional manner," I replied.

As Senior Move Managers, we sometimes worked with individuals who were already emotionally fragile and then put them under the added stress of preparing for a move. This family had been fragile and unhealthy for a long time. We hadn't caused the issues they were struggling with, and we could not fix them. Their house, with all its memories, was toxic to their relationship. A new environment might help them start over, but there was no way to circumvent the pain they were experiencing. As professionals, we did our part by listening compassionately and helping them achieve their goals. Although we did our best to mitigate the stress of moving, some people are like china that's been repaired: they are just too fragile. Some things can't be mended.

Although moving and childbirth are both challenging, most people willingly do them not because we forget the pain, but because they are worth it. Most people believe the joy of having children outweighs the pain of childbirth, and in spite of the many challenges of downsizing and moving, most older adults who relocate are happy with the outcome. That's why I hope this couple was able to move on once they left the home where their son died. Although there are no guarantees their life would be better in a new environment, the move represented possibility. Staying put, there was none.

I vote for possibility.

In spite of the many challenges of downsizing and moving, most older adults who relocate are happy with the outcome.

22

Fear of Abandonment

We all fear emotional abandonment. No one wants to feel undesired, left behind, discarded. The death of people we love creates a feeling of abandonment, but over time, healing takes place. Not so for abandonment by friends while we are still alive.

In his blog Watching the Lights Go Out, *retired physician David Hilfiker wrote about his emotions after being diagnosed with early-stage dementia. As a physician, Hilfiker understood the course of the disease all too well, but the disease itself was not his biggest fear. His biggest fear was shame and abandonment. He anticipated what others would think of him and how they would react because he knew what he thought and how he reacted to people with dementia. "What do I say to him? How do I respond when he asks me my name for the fourth time in fifteen minutes or repeats a story he just told us?"*

Because of his discomfort, Hilfiker would find some way to abandon the person with dementia, not because he wanted to, but because he didn't know what else to do.[1]

But then tables were turned, and Hilfiker was the one in danger of being abandoned. In his blog, Hilfiker wants those who don't have Alzheimer's disease to understand what it's like to be in his position, "so you can allow yourself to find your way into the world of the Alzheimer's disease sufferer, find your way back into relationship and won't have to abandon me or others so easily."

This had such an impact on me. When I thought of all that Alzheimer's disease represents, it never occurred to me that abandonment would be one of the biggest fears.

I intended to order a book from BookBub that I vaguely remembered as a film comedy starring Hugh Grant—*Four Weddings and a Funeral*. Instead, I ordered a book titled *Four Funerals and a Wedding*. It was very different from what I expected.[2]

Four Funerals and a Wedding, by Jill Smolowe, is a book about resilience. A fifty-something woman talks about the deaths of her husband, sister, mother, and mother-in-law—all in fifteen months. God willing, most of us won't go through that much loss in so short a time, but many of us will go through that much loss over our lives.

In spite of its title, *Four Funerals and a Wedding* is not about dying. It's about living through loss and developing your unique perspective on how to deal with grief. Smolowe emphasizes that there is no formula for how to behave.

Although Smolowe feels abandoned by the deaths of her loved ones, the story that most stood out for me was her fear of abandonment by those still living. She remembers how she avoided a recently widowed woman because she didn't know what to say and wonders if friends are avoiding her for the same reason. Smolowe's situation is very different from Hilfiker's, yet they share a fear of abandonment.

Jill also talks about how people react when you share bad news. Some give advice. Some insist on discussing personal issues or issues that may not be a priority to you. Most don't know what to say. But some, and these were the ones she especially valued, simply asked how could they help.

I wasn't sure what I thought about this book, but when a friend wrote recently that tests showed ominous "hot spots," I thought about the lesson I learned and asked simply, "How can I help?"

Thanks to people like Hilfiker, Smolowe, and others who fearlessly describe what it feels like to be emotionally abandoned, we have reminders of how to be better versions of ourselves. This just goes to show: sometimes you don't get the book you want, you get the book you need.

Once we're at a certain age, we're likely to have friends going through serious illness as well as friends experiencing the loss of loved ones. Like it or not, we need to figure out how to respond to them, how to be a friend. We need to figure out how not to abandon them because of our own emotional discomfort. It's messy, and we may bungle it sometimes, but perfection is not required.

Like it or not, we need to figure out how to respond to them, how to be a friend. We need to figure out how not to abandon them because of our own emotional discomfort.

Many people find it hard to ask for help, especially when they are most hurting. I know I felt that way when my husband, Bill, had a serious heart attack two years ago. When I was feeling overwhelmed, stripped of resources, and naked in my neediness, simply being asked, "How can I help?" provided more comfort than you can imagine.

23

Caregiving

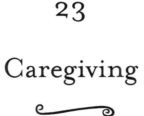

According to psychotherapist Maud Purcell, adult children are unprepared for the roller coaster of emotions they experience as their parents age. Those who view their parents' lives as characterized by pervasive loss have an especially hard time.[1]

One day I overheard a conversation.

"How are your parents doing?" one asked.

"Oh, you know, they're deteriorating," said the other.

That's it? I thought. That's how she sums up her parents . . . they're deteriorating? What about "They're facing some challenges, but they're coping," or "They're declining and struggling to maintain their independence," or "All things considered, they're pretty resilient." Almost anything was better than reducing her parents to a short description of passive diminishment—they're deteriorating.

And that's when I thought about my dog.

Poppy is an old dog, very old for a greyhound. Her regal face is mostly white, and her deep brown eyes that once reached into your soul when she stared at you are clouded with cataracts. The muscles in her once-powerful hind legs are atrophied. That, combined with arthritis, makes transitions from surfaces difficult for her. Often she needs help getting into bed, steadying herself on stairs, or getting up from a nap. She has lost weight, so her ribs are prominent, even for a greyhound. Her coat sheds constantly. Her failing kidneys cause her to drink more, and this in turn results in numerous accidents in the house since she can't move fast enough to get outside. She takes a long time to respond to simple commands, like "come," which we attribute to a combination of slower mental processing speed, hearing impairment, and mobility issues. She sleeps most of the day and tires quickly. Although we care for Poppy, we get little back from her compared to the funny, affectionate dog she once was. We don't ask her to be who she once was, because we are okay with who she is now. If asked how Poppy is doing, I would say, "Poppy is an old dog, but she's doing great." I would never say, "She's deteriorating."

Similarly, we had no sadness caring for Tiger, our twenty-one-year-old cat. When we noticed physical changes in Tiger, we implemented a series of aging-in-place modifications so he could remain independent and injury-free. These included a three-step pet ladder, so Tiger could get on and off my husband's chair. When Tiger could no longer navigate the five-inch-high walls of the litter box, we cut a new entrance into it with a one-inch-high lip. We built steps into our sunroom so Tiger could continue going outside, and brushed him daily when he could no longer groom himself. When failing kidneys caused him to drink large quantities of water, we changed the litter box daily and spread paper around it, because he often missed the box entirely. We weren't just concerned for Tiger's independence; we were concerned for his dignity.

My husband asked if I would take as good care of him when he aged. We laughed, but it gave me pause. Why is it so much easier to care for beloved pets as they age than for beloved people? The physical tasks we performed for Tiger and Poppy were unglamorous and sometimes distasteful, but they were not an unwelcome burden. We were not angry, frustrated, or resentful, yet people often express these feelings when caring for elderly family members. Aging pets bring out the best in us. We are caring, compassionate, resilient, and resourceful. We accept aging pets for who they are and are not saddened by how changed they are from their younger selves. Mostly, we experience joy in their existence and are happy for every day we have with them.

Caregiving for elderly family members is rocky terrain, but there is opportunity for richness and rewarding experiences as well. Maybe old dogs can teach us new tricks after all.

When I age, I want to be like Tiger. I want to be as independent as possible and live in an environment that maximizes my dignity and minimizes my impairments. I want to be surrounded by people who accept me for who I am, even though

I am different from who I once was. I want a good quality of life, where I can continue to do the things that are important to me. And like Tiger, I want to give love as well as receive it.

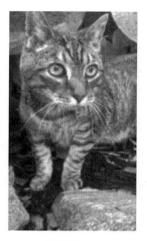

RIP Tiger

24

Plan B

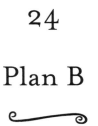

In his 1962 State of the Union address, John Kennedy said, "The time to repair the roof is when the sun is shining." [1] Great concept; that's Plan A. Plan B is to buy a tarp.

In popular language, Plan B is the alternate plan in case the first plan (Plan A) fails. In short, Plan B is second best. I think Plan B gets a bad rap; there is a lot to be said for Plan B.

Take the client whose house sells more quickly than expected and who needs to live in temporary housing for several weeks or months until their new apartment is available. The client groans at the thought of moving twice (Plan B) until I remind her that having a home sell for a price she wanted, not going through weeks of living in a home while keeping it market-ready, and not having the anxiety of waiting and wondering if the house would sell is a good problem to have.

Plan B, living with things in storage for a few weeks or months, ends up being a good plan. Ironically, when these clients finally move into their permanent home, having spent weeks or months with things in storage, they realize they did fine with a lot less around them. When their things come out of storage, they willingly part with items they had previously thought essential.

Take the husband who says, "I've been caregiving for my wife 24/7 for five years and I'm used up." He's being clear that he's maxed out and cannot handle the added stress of preparing to move while also caring for his wife. Conventional wisdom (Plan A) is to sort through and dispose of everything not going with him before the move. But the best solution for this man is Plan B, which reduces his stress by minimizing his pre-move involvement.

With Plan B, he selects a small number of things to go immediately to the apartment, and everything else stays in the old house, to be dealt with later. After the move, when his wife is being cared for by others, he returns to the house, better equipped physically and emotionally to deal with the items not taken.

Plan A says do it right the first time. Plan B says do what works. In a perfect world, they are one and the same, but the world is seldom perfect.

Plan A and Plan B are both about moving forward, but they use different approaches to make progress. The best approach depends on many factors—personality, situation, timing.

Sometimes the decision between Plan A or Plan B is based on pragmatism. Take paper, for example. Many people have piles of paper in every room: mail, insurance forms, receipts, paid and unpaid bills, lists, notes, investment records, coupons. Plan A is to sort, shred, and dispose of papers before the move. Plan A is logical but not realistic. If they could easily sort and organize papers, there wouldn't be piles of paper everywhere. Instead of focusing on what's clearly a struggle for them, Plan B is to pack the piles into boxes and deal with them after the move.

Sometimes, the decision between Plan A or Plan B is based on perspective.

I met with a client in her early eighties who had lost her husband and then, a few months later, suffered a stroke. They had planned to move to a nearby senior living community, and my client wanted to continue with that plan. As she recuperated from the stroke and dealt with the loss of her husband, planning for the new villa gave her purpose. She worked with a decorator and implemented changes that made the villa her own. She was looking forward to the move.

Plan A says do it right the first time. Plan B says do what works. In a perfect world, they are one and the same, but the world is seldom perfect.

Shortly before her move date, my client was evaluated to see if she could resume driving and did not pass. Without the ability to drive, her children argued, moving to a villa was a mistake. It would be harder to join activities, and there would be fewer opportunities to socialize. Wouldn't it be better to move to an apartment in the main building? That was her children's Plan A.

The client saw things differently. In less than a year, she'd lost her husband, her health, her ability to drive, and her home of forty years. The villa was something to move toward, something in which she had invested time, energy, and passion. To my client, moving to the villa was Plan A. I hoped her children would support her decision, and fortunately, they did.

I saw this dynamic reenacted repeatedly when frail clients chose to move to independent living. "Why not move directly into assisted living so there is just one move?" their children would ask.

"Because the move to independent living is the move your parents are willing to make," I would respond. "Faced with the choice of moving to assisted living now or remaining in the family home, your parents will likely choose to remain in their home. If they move to independent living and soon need more care, the second move will be easier because they will already be in the community they call home."

Sometimes I compared it to sailing. Sailing downwind is easy; you can mostly head in the direction you want to go. But to sail upwind, you need to tack against the wind. Tacking is the concept of making progress by zigzagging rather than moving forward directly. Faced with formidable obstacles, going sideways is sometimes the best way to move forward. This is true in sailing, and in life.

In 279 B.C.E., King Pyrrhus of Epirus defeated the Romans at Asculum but lost his best officers and many of his men. As the armies separated and Pyrrhus was congratulated on his victory, he replied, "One other such victory would utterly undo me." Thus was born the concept of a Pyrrhic victory—a victory that inflicts such a devastating toll on the victor that it is tantamount to defeat.

Early in my career as a Senior Move Manager, I heard the phrase Pyrrhic victory and was struck by its applicability to my work with older adults and their families. Sometimes, Plan A requires a level of commitment, effort, or compromise that is so high that the value of winning is questionable. Sometimes zigzagging is the best way to move forward. That's why Plan B is my plan of choice. Not because it is lesser or easier.

●────────●

Plan B is where experience meets reality and comes up with a solution.

25

Gifts with Strings

In 1985, when my husband and I renovated our home, my mother-in-law, Bubbie (who you met in Part 1), offered us $200 to buy a microwave. We did not own a microwave at that time and were certain we didn't want one. "If we don't get a microwave, she'll still give us the $200, right?" I asked my husband.

"Absolutely," he said.

He was wrong. The offer was a microwave or nothing. So that is how I got my first microwave—but it wasn't my first gift with strings.

Gifts with strings are gifts we give to someone else but with conditions attached. I remember a client who had a Henredon burled mahogany highboy that wouldn't fit in her new home. Burled woods are rare and hard to work with; they're considered luxurious. She offered the highboy to her children and was delighted when her daughter wanted it as a bureau for the woman's granddaughter. A few months later, my client visited her daughter and went to her granddaughter's room to look at the highboy. There it was—painted blue. At first, she was aghast. They had painted a burled mahogany highboy. Then she realized she had to "zip it." She had given the highboy away.

This makes perfect sense intellectually, but we don't give things away with our brains, we give them away with our hearts, and our hearts don't let go.

My ninety-one-year-old Aunt Betty, on the other hand, planned to retain control of her gifts. Married three times, she had a lot of diamond rings. Three decades ago, she confided that she didn't plan to leave the rings to me. "You have a son," she explained. (I have two sons and a daughter, but, unlike me, Betty never considered my stepchildren to be my children.) "And when he grows up, he may find a girl and want to get married and need a ring. But then he may get divorced and the ring would leave the family, so I am giving the rings to Miriam."

Miriam, my niece, was at that time seven years old. As years passed, I did not have the heart to tell my aunt that Miriam, now grown, was seeing someone seriously. She might get married, and I think they want children. One

> ... we don't give things away with our brains, we give them away with our hearts, and our hearts don't let go.

of those children could be a boy, and when he grows up, he might meet a girl, want to get married, and need a ring ... My aunt planned to control what happened to those rings in this life and the next.

When my grandmother offered me things, she expected me to accept, keep, and use them, and I did keep them, even if that meant storing a sterling silver bread dish in the basement for forty years. I think most people my age accepted these obligations, these strings, when we received gifts, but we are the last generation to be controlled by guilt. Our children have no problem rejecting our gifts or changing or disposing of them once they're given.

In his book *Downsizing: Confronting Our Possessions in Later Life*, David J. Ekerdt describes how satisfying it is to dispose of items with safe passage—giving them a good home where the item will be protected, create legacy, or benefit the recipient. [1]

Creating safe passage with family members is messy, because often we don't truly relinquish gifts we give. We attach strings that lead to resentment or disappointment for both giver and recipient. As a generation of Boomers prepares to downsize, it's not just our possessions we need to deal with. We need to prepare ourselves emotionally to let go so we don't give gifts with strings.

26

The Ethics of
Geriatric Fiblets

The term "geriatric fiblet" was coined at the 2000 World Alzheimer's Congress as "necessary white lies to redirect loved ones or discourage them from detrimental behavior." [1] It was primarily directed at working with individuals who have dementia. Is it appropriate to use geriatric fiblets with people who do not have dementia? I think it is. Sometimes, it's not about competency; it's about independence, dignity, and kindness.

The senior move management industry is guided by a code of ethics that defines the values and principles of behavior for the profession. Developed in 2002 by the National Association of Senior Move Managers (NASMM), the code includes client confidentiality, honoring the client's right to determine their own future, respecting the client's belongings, acting with integrity, and more. (You can view the entire code of ethics on www.NASMM.org).[2]

Do family members have different standards than professionals working with older adults? I think they do. As I looked back at my career as a Senior Move Manager, I reflected on this question.

Scenario 1

Take, for example, a client who has 100 *National Geographic* magazines. He doesn't want to keep them but doesn't want them thrown away either. "Can't you find someone who wants them?" he asks. A friend who teaches third grade agrees to take half the magazines for an art project. I give her half, recycle the rest, and inform my client, "I found a third-grade teacher who is using the magazines in an art project." I tell the truth, sort of, except I omit the detail that half the magazines were discarded. In short, I tell a fiblet. As a Senior Move Manager, this fiblet is one I can live with. I think it shows respect for my client's wishes.

Scenario 2

An adult daughter is sorting through her parents' belongings, much of which will not fit in their new home. "Throw this away and don't tell my parents," she tells me. "Say you never saw it." The daughter may tell this fiblet to her parents, but I will not. According to the NASMM code of ethics, my clients determine what goes with them to their new home, not their children. My responsibility is to provide guidance but respect my clients' decisions, even if I don't agree with them. On the other hand, when I helped my aunt move, I discarded her worn out underwear. At that time, I was acting as a family member, not as a Move Manager.

More complex is when the daughter throws something out without asking her parents and then asks me not to tell her parents. Am I obligated to blow the whistle on the daughter? The code of ethics says I should promote cooperation among individuals involved in the client's move. Sharing the daughter's conversation would cause major family disruption. How do you decide what to do when options seem in conflict? In this case, I looked at context and at the emotional cost of each course of action. I opted for family unity and kept silent about the daughter's behavior.

Scenario 3

What about adult children who ask me to tell their parents my fees are lower than they are, while the children make up the difference in secret? I recognize they are trying to respect their parents' desire for independence. As a Senior Move Manager, my relationship with my client is built on trust. I would decline to lie about my fees. On the other hand, thirty years ago, I orchestrated this exact scenario for my grandmother. Anya was determined to pay no more than $200 per month for an apartment, but the apartment she wanted was $260 a month. We asked the leasing agent if we could pay the difference. "No problem," she replied, and she prepared a dummy lease. Amazingly, my grandmother accepted that she was being given a discount because "her deceased son had been a doctor," and she agreed not to discuss her special deal with other residents.

I had no qualms about participating in this rental fee deception. I was acting as a family member, and my fiblet enabled my grandmother to preserve her dignity and independence. As a family member, my actions were guided by love and expediency. As a Move Manager, my actions are guided by a code of ethics.

We all tell fiblets, especially to people we love and whose feelings we care about, whether they are parents, spouses, or children. "White lies are extremely common in healthy relationships," says licensed psychologist and relationship expert Susan Orenstein, Ph.D. Orenstein defines white lies as "omitting the complete truth to spare someone's feelings." The main consideration in determining when to tell a white lie, experts say, is to ask yourself who benefits from the lie—the person lying or the person being lied to? Is lying the kinder communication and the best alternative? [3]

But even with family members, this issue is controversial. Like many things worth thinking about, it's complicated.

27

The Upside of Risk

In simple terms, risk involves uncertainty about the effects of an activity. Most people associate risk with undesirable consequences. Geriatrician Bill Thomas says we're only seeing half the picture—the downside of risk. "Risk also includes the possibility that things will turn out better than expected," says Thomas. "When we remove the downside of risk, we remove the upside of risk as well." This is especially prevalent in long-term care, where the imperative to minimize downside risk has minimized upside risk as well. Thomas argues that life should include a balance between upside and downside risk, because that is where richness, independence, and possibility reside. [1]

What helped me truly understand this concept was a dog.

I met a woman and her dog walking along a nature trail. As dog lovers do, we started to talk. She said she and her dog walk the two-mile nature trail daily. Recently, she told me, she tried to adopt a five-year-old dog, to keep her other dog company, but was turned down. Since she was seventy-six, the rescue organization said it was likely something would happen to her during the dog's lifetime and the dog would need to be rehomed. Rather than put the dog's future at risk, they rejected the woman's application. This is what I call the tail wagging the dog.

> ... life should include a balance between upside and downside risk, because that is where richness, independence, and possibility reside.

The numerous benefits that accrue to older pet owners are well documented. Pets reduce stress, lower blood pressure, and increase physical activity. They provide companionship, reduce depression, increase social interactions, and decrease loneliness. Senior pet owners visit the doctor less often, have fewer minor health problems, lower medical costs, better psychological well-being, and even higher survival rates following surgery. Pets do more than bring joy to older pet owners; they provide purpose.[2]

There are downside risks for older pet owners as well. Pets can have unexpected expenses, contribute to trips and falls, create messes that need to be cleaned up and die, leaving their owners heartbroken. Of these, falls are the most concerning. Older adults have worse balance, and are more likely to trip on a pet and be seriously injured if they do. For older adults especially, falls can be life changing. Nevertheless, most older pet owners believe the upside risks of pet ownership—the social, mental, and health benefits—more than outweigh the downside risks and willingly bring pets into their lives.

What about risk for the dog? Pets who are adopted by older adults are lucky! Older adopters have lots of time to devote to previously unwanted pets, much more time than younger adopters who are working or busy with childcare duties. These pets go from the pound to paradise. Both pets and people benefit when older adults adopt pets.

The pet rescue organization looked at the risk/benefit paradigm differently. They ignored upside risk for the dog and focused on downside risk only. The woman I met walking was a vigorous, healthy seventy-six-year-old who exercised daily. They rejected her application based on age alone, as if every seventy-six-year-old is the same. It's true that health can change quickly at seventy-six, but life situations change quickly at any age, whether it's a new job, a divorce, an illness, or a move from a house to an apartment.

Armed with good intentions, the rescue organization tried to control what would happen to the animals they adopted out, but no one can control the future. Animals have a right to the upside of risk, just as humans do. If there is essence to a dog's soul, it is having purpose and making a difference in its owner's life, and that is what animals do for elderly pet owners. Perhaps those dogs do have a higher risk of needing to be rehomed, but that is a risk most dogs would gladly accept (were they able) in exchange for a life filled with love and purpose.

Bill Thomas's theory of upside and downside risk was developed in response to the widespread practice in health care of surplus safety—reducing risk at all costs. But its application extends to our own lives as well. My husband and I covet time at our shore home but faced significant consequences when he needed urgent medical care and we were several hours from major medical centers. Yet we happily return to the shore. We are willing to assume the downside of risk, being far from optimal medical care, because we value the upside of risk, the beauty of living on the water. It's a decision that we, as independent and cognitively intact adults, can make. Some people may disagree with our choices, but they likely agree with our right to make them. At least, they agree at this point in our lives. What if we become frail or cognitively impaired? When will we lose the right to make decisions, good or bad, about how we want to live?

When I was a Senior Move Manager, I met with an eighty-nine-year-old man who hoarded. I'll call him Dr. F. A retired dentist, Dr. F. lived alone in a five-bedroom house, in which every room was filled with stuff. In the kitchen, there was an eighteen-inch aisle to walk through. He had no access to his sink or stove and received home-delivered meals. None of the bedrooms could be entered because they were filled to the ceiling and the doors could not be opened. He slept on a cot in the basement. His living room, dining room, hallways, garage, and basement were similarly accessed by narrow aisles. Every horizontal surface in the house was occupied.

After we toured his home, we stood in his foyer and chatted. Dr. F. was aware that his behavior was considered to be hoarding. He had read numerous articles about hoarding and talked about the Collyer Brothers, two eccentric men in New York City who suffocated when the tons of paper and debris in their home fell on them.[3]

I suggested a plan to make one room in his house—the den next to the kitchen—a space he could sit. It was a modest goal. I was not trying to change him or clear out his home; I just wanted to provide one area where he could sit and talk to someone. To remove money as a barrier to using our services, I offered several sorting sessions at no charge. My hope was that he would experience working with us and develop trust. Dr. F. seemed to truly enjoy my visit. I believed he was lonely and would have been happy having people to talk to regardless of what got accomplished during the sessions.

Repeatedly, however, Dr. F. turned me down. "I know what hoarding has cost me in terms of connections to people," he said. "I know I might fall and that for people my age, falls can be life-threatening. But this is how I live. I'm doing pretty well for eighty-nine. I haven't fallen yet, and I hope I don't, but that is a risk I am willing to live with."

Given his age and degree of hoarding, Dr. F.'s hoarding behavior posed a significant risk. Did that mean it was appropriate for social service organizations to intervene? At eighty-nine, had Dr. F. lost his right to make decisions about how he lived?

We all take risks, and we all make bad decisions at times. Some of us smoke, some of us are non-compliant with medications, some of us are overweight, some of us postpone mammograms, many of us talk or text on phones while driving. Like Dr. F., we know the potential consequences, and yet, we still choose to assume risk every day. I don't want my right to assume risk—both downside and upside—taken away, and neither did Dr. F.

28

Downsizing Revisited

Two years ago, my husband and I bought a second home. It was our dream come true. We wanted "lock and leave," so we could get to the new home easily, so we decided to move to a senior living community. We were downsizing our possessions so we could upsize our lives. The timing was perfect. What could go wrong?

Three months before our move date, my husband had a planned hip placement. Two days later, he had a massive heart attack. In the blink of an eye, we went from moving under the best of circumstances to moving under the worst of circumstances.

I never considered not moving. Bill could not return to our three-story colonial.

Because I had been a professional Senior Move Manager, I knew exactly what to do to have a seamless, stress-free move. I started downsizing early and made great progress. A lot didn't come with us, but a lot did. When I look at things that made the cut, I see themes.

Some things made the cut because of rationalization . . . like our thirty-cup coffee urn. "I might have a large dinner party," I rationalized. Never mind that I hadn't used the coffee urn in six years. I might need it.

Some things made the cut because of procrastination, like five outdoor hoses that arrived at our new home. I had meant to cull them and select the best one but ran out of time. Not that it required much time; I just didn't get to it. So on move day, I told the movers, "Just take them all."

Some things made the cut for no logical reason, like a bag filled with panty hose I had worn in my corporate days, twenty-five years earlier. I'm not sure how the bag survived in my closet without being culled, let alone made it to the senior living community, but it's here.

Some things made the cut because I was pragmatic, like four cartons of photo albums. Sorting through photos takes time. Even if we succeeded in eliminating half of the photos, it would only reduce our load by two cartons. There were sixty cartons of other things in the basement that needed to be gone before moving, and I knew I could deal with all sixty in less time than it would take to sort through the photos. That's why four cartons of photos came with us to our cottage, but sixty cartons of other stuff did not.

Some things made the cut because they were emotional, like my mom's set of Rosenthal china. Service for sixteen, it was my mom's pride and joy. It has a delicate floral print, which means it can't go in the dishwasher, and a gold rim, which means it can't go in the microwave. In the forty years since my mom died, I've taken good care of her dishes. I stored them in my basement. Now they're stored in the garage of my cottage. I'm not sure I've truly honored my mom by keeping her dishes in cartons for four decades, but they're here.

Some things made the cut because they were logical in my old home . . . they're just not logical in my new home. Like our stained-glass lamps. Our old home was dark with no overhead lighting, so it needed a lot of lamps. Our cottage is light-filled with lots of overhead lighting. I placed a favorite lamp where it always stood, on the round table next to my husband's chair. On that table it competes for space with a box of tissues, his coffee mug, three remotes, throat lozenges, and his iPad. Light in our new home is so much better that in the time we've lived here, we've never once turned the lamp on. Bringing the lamp was logical, but keeping it isn't.

So what did the move of a professional downsizer look like? It was far from perfect. It included rationalization, procrastination, and pragmatism. It included decisions that were emotional and sometimes illogical. Some decisions have since been remade, some not, and it doesn't matter. In spite of all the imperfections, we're moved in and enjoying our new life.

I learned some important lessons along the way.

I learned that perfection in downsizing is not required. If things made the cut that shouldn't have, it wasn't the end of the world. I could deal with them later.

I learned not to delay moving until timing is perfect. Our timing was perfect, and then it was horrible, but it all turned out okay.

I learned that despite careful planning, life is unpredictable, and perfection is not required. If I wait for perfection, I might postpone relationships and experiences that could enrich my life.

———————

People don't have to be whole to have value, endings don't have to be perfect, and solutions are often not black and white. Life (and death) are messy, lines blur, and amidst all this imperfection, there is opportunity for greatness.

PART 5

Planting Trees

❧

"A society grows great when
old men plant trees whose shade they
know they shall never sit in."
–ANCIENT PROVERB

Susan Bosak of the Legacy Project asks, "Where do you think it's best to plant a young tree: a clearing in an old-growth forest or in an open field?" Ecologists tell us that young trees grow better when they are planted in an area with older trees. The reason is that the roots of the young tree are able to follow pathways created by former trees and implant themselves more deeply. Over time, the roots of some trees actually graft themselves to one another, creating an intricate, interdependent foundation. Stronger trees share resources with weaker ones so that the whole forest becomes healthier. [1] That's a way to describe legacy—an interconnection across time, where those who have come before us take responsibility for those who come after.

Over the years, I've met many people who planted trees. They created legacy, ritual, and meaning for themselves, for their family, and for future generations. These are their stories.

29

Creating Legacy

I have decided to make a former client my role model. I met him half a dozen years ago, when he was in his early eighties and moving to a senior living community. As we began planning his move, he said, "I lost my wife three years ago. Sorting through our belongings makes me feel like I'm losing her all over again—I wish I could go away and come back after the move."

So, rather than be present at the move, he attended a conference across the country and became our first "I'd rather go on vacation" moving client. Since then, I have thought often about his ability to articulate his feelings and, faced with an emotional challenge, his willingness to take a course of action that worked for him.

I met him again several years later and learned that he had moved to a different apartment within the community to be near a woman he had met. "She introduced me to the literary club," he said. "It consists of five women and me. We meet every Thursday before dinner. We laugh, drink, and talk about no literature.

"She is a very interesting woman, an artist," he continued. "Her apartment is across the hall from mine. The door to her apartment has a sign: 'Outrageous older woman lives here.'"

He introduced me to her. She used a wheelchair, was full of life, and was wonderfully memorable. I was happy for him.

My client was the former director of a multi-hospital system and a pioneer in the then-nascent industry of hospital administration. Then in his early eighties, he taught in a graduate program he had helped found at a nearby university and lunched regularly with current and former grad students. Before I left, he confided, "This move [to the senior living community] has so exceeded my expectations. I never expected my ninth decade to be so rewarding."

I met with my former client again a year later. Sadly, his friend the artist had passed away. He was on his way to the community's chess club, where he and other members (all over eighty) met regularly with the chess club of an inner-city high school. They were helping the kids get ready for a city-wide tournament. He was also preparing for the second half of an oral history project conducted by the American Hospital Association. In recognition of his pioneering leadership role in hospital administration, he explained, they had interviewed him in 1980 and wanted to meet with him again, three decades later, to discuss his perspective on how the industry had evolved. In preparation, he was reviewing his professional accomplishments.

> I never expected my ninth decade to be so rewarding.

The oral history people have it all wrong, I thought to myself. What's important here is not his contribution to the health care industry (although it was considerable); it's the way he lives his life now. When I am older, I hope I'll have the same comments about my ninth decade, that I will form new, meaningful relationships, laugh, be engaged with community, and give back to others. As a Senior Move Manager, I helped thousands of people downsize. Many considered possessions to be their legacy. To me, a legacy is not something you leave; it's something you make. My client made a great legacy. I hope I can do the same.

⌒

Some people create legacy as a natural continuation of their life's path. Others stumble upon a concept that captivates and revitalizes them. So it was for Mr. S., an accountant from Broomall, Pennsylvania. One day, Mr. S. saw a documentary at his synagogue, and his life changed forever.[1]

> Many considered possessions to be their legacy. To me, a legacy is not something you leave; it's something you make.

The documentary was about a middle school in Whitwell, Tennessee that started a Holocaust education program to teach children about tolerance. The children had difficulty comprehending the massive scale of the Holocaust, and began collecting paperclips to represent the human lives lost. After a slow start, an article about the project appeared in the *Washington Post*[2] and millions of paper clips started arriving at the school, often accompanied by stories or a dedication to someone who had died during the Holocaust. An authentic German rail car used to transport Jews to concentration camps was donated to the school and became part of the Children's Holocaust Memorial, which was located on school grounds. Three years later, the documentary *Paper Clips* was released, describing how a project to teach tolerance in a tiny Appalachian town where not a single Jew lived, became a catalyst that changed lives within and beyond the town. [3]

Smitten by the story of Whitwell, Mr. S. wanted to thank those involved, so he and his wife made the 800-mile trip from Philadelphia with notes written by students in the synagogue's Hebrew school describing how the movie had moved them. "They gave us a personal tour of the school and the rail car," said Mr. S. "It was an emotional, change-of-life moment for me, and I realized I had a project for life." A few years later, he funded design and construction of a 9-ft paperclip mounted in front of his Broomall synagogue on two tons of Jerusalem stone, imported from Israel.

I heard about this story when I moved Mr. S. and his wife to a senior living community. His passion and excitement about his legacy remained unabated.

In the process of enriching their own lives, these clients enriched the lives of many others. To me, their stories embody the concept of legacy—roots grafting onto roots that came before them, creating interconnectedness and a stronger foundation for the future.

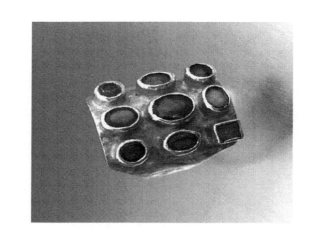

30

Creating Legacy
Through Objects

D ividing family possessions can be a source of struggle, as it was with my brother Michael and me, but for many, it can be a source of meaningful discussion. Workbooks like *Who Gets Grandma's Yellow Pie Plate* provide templates for discussions about dividing personal property among family members in a positive way. [1]

I think the biggest determinant of how family members deal with belongings after a death is their existing relationship. Michael and I had a poor relationship while my mom was alive, so it's not surprising that we argued about what would happen to her things after she died. For family members who have good relationships, dividing possessions after a death can be creative, elegant, and meaningful. When this occurs, the items themselves aren't the legacy; the way they are dealt with becomes the legacy.

After their mom died, two sisters, who were friends of mine, couldn't decide who would get two special items they both wanted. One was a sterling silver pitcher their mother purchased at an auction when the girls were young. The pitcher had an ornate letter "F" engraved on it. Their mom must have been omniscient because years later, both girls married men whose last names began with "F." Some things are too strange to ponder.

The other item was a beautiful ring their mother purchased on a shopping trip to New York City.

Neither sister could choose one item over the other, so they developed a plan to share them, and over the years, added their own traditions. The ring was always worn on New Year's Eve, and the pitcher was always returned to the other sister with fresh flowers in it on New Year's Day. The ring, whose photo appears at the beginning of this chapter, is a wearable memory, an intimate, personal way of staying connected with their mother throughout the year. The pitcher is a physical presence displayed proudly in both homes. Both objects lead to stories about their mom, the coincidence about the letter F, and the ritual they started in order to share the two items.

I love how the sisters handled this because their solution is about relationship, not ownership. Their ritual celebrates loving memories of their mom as well as the good relationship between the siblings. It's a wonderful legacy to pass on to the next generation.

Between them, my friends have five children, four girls and a boy. The sisters assume they will need to decide who keeps the ring and who keeps the pitcher, since when they die, getting agreement among five cousins and spouses will be more complex than it was between two sisters. I like to think that their

> . . . their solution is about relationship, not ownership.

children will find a way to continue the tradition. They have a good start; their parents have given them a great role model.

My brother Mark and I do something similar with a needlepoint chair that belonged to my mother. Some years the chair lives at my house and some years at his. For me, the chair is a physical symbol of the good relationship I have with Mark and Sue, my sister-in-law. Of all the things my mother left me, I think my relationship with Mark is the legacy she would be most proud of, and that's the legacy I'll pass on to my kids.

Recently, I heard of another way objects were being used to create legacy. Instead of passing down objects from the past, some people have begun to take an object from the present and transform it into a meaningful ritual that celebrates new connections while preserving those from the past.

It started several years ago, at a Passover Seder, but it could occur at any family event. My friend took a new tablecloth and asked each person at the Seder to sign their name. She then embroidered the names on the tablecloth. The following year, the same tablecloth was used. One guest had passed away since the last Seder, and their name on the tablecloth was a way of keeping them at the table. New guests were asked to sign their name, and these were later embroidered as well. They are starting the third year of this tradition, and already her children have selected the tablecloth as something they want to have "when they grow up." My friend took an ordinary item that had no special meaning and transformed it, creating a ritual that celebrates family and friends and evolves over time. Her legacy combines connection and tradition, looks backwards and forwards, is inclusive and simple. It's perfect.

PART 6

Possibility

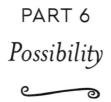

Judy moved into the senior living community in summer. Glenn moved in six months later. There was nothing to indicate they were meant to be together. Judy, divorced twice, was petite, vivacious, and outgoing. Glenn, a recent widower, was tall, thin, and quiet. An artist, Judy was energized by variety and moved seamlessly from one medium to another. An accountant, Glenn's work life was constant and consistent. Meeting by chance in the exercise room, outgoing Judy smiled at Glenn, and shy Glenn smiled back. They chatted, and then chatted some more. They soon became friends, and then more than friends. Asked who initiated the first kiss, Judy responded she had, but added, "Glenn moved quickly after that." Months later, they married and moved into the same apartment.

Judy and Glenn enjoy an active life and do most things together, including a tender afternoon nap. Reflecting on their new life, they marvel at finding love in their ninth decade. When asked if the word that best describes their relationship is hope, Judy thought for a moment and replied, "No, it's possibility."

Hope—the belief that something can or will happen—feels aspirational, a potential result that may or may not happen, and that does not require action by you.

Possibility is also about what may or may not happen, but possibility implies responsibility to take an active role in creating the result you want. With hope and possibility, there are no guarantees, but with possibility there is the ability to participate, to have a role in controlling the future. Put another way, I hope that I will win the lottery. If I buy a ticket, there is a possibility it will happen.

> There is much richness to be had in the second half of life, but we need to buy a ticket.

This last section is about possibility in the second half of life. There is much richness to be had in the second half of life, but we need to buy a ticket.

31

The Art of Connection

One day about fifteen years ago, I went to get a haircut and came home with a tattoo. I had never considered it before and can't tell you why I did it. My husband, who had gotten his first tattoo at age sixty, was delighted; my friends were horrified. I didn't care! I was part of the growing trend of senior ink.

Tattoos, now considered a form of body art, have long been an example of self-expression. There are many reasons why people get tattoos, but for older adults, a big part of getting a tattoo is the experience. "It made me feel sort of adventurous and wild," said tattooed eighty-five-year-old Helen Lambin, of Chicago.[1] That's how it made me feel, too. It had been a long time since I did anything wild or spontaneous. Getting a tattoo made me feel alive.

Today, 5 percent of people getting their first tattoo are over sixty, and 15 percent of baby boomers have

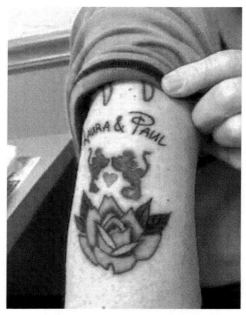

My brother-in-law Paul's tattoo
that says Laura and Paul.

tattoos. A decade earlier, these figures were close to zero.[2] Some people cite the change in societal attitudes as giving them more freedom to express themselves through ink. Others credit life stage. Since many folks over sixty are already retired, "You'll never get a decent job," is no longer a concern. Neither is, "You'll regret it later when you're old and your skin sags." Their skin already sags. One woman said her mother forbade her, saying, "Over my dead body." Her mother is now dead. As people get older, they become more comfortable with themselves and are less influenced by what others think about them. Maybe it's simply being more comfortable in their own skin.

The aspect of senior ink that most intrigues me is that senior tattoos are less about personal expression and more about connection. Helen Lambin says tattoos are how she makes friends. "With my tattoos, I get to talk to people I wouldn't normally get the chance to meet."

Five years ago, my brother-in-law Paul informed his five grandchildren that if any of them wanted to get a tattoo, Pop-Pop would get one with them. So far, three of his grandchildren have taken him up on his offer, and he has flown around the country to be with them. Mickey and Minnie, seen in the photo, were created in Boise, Idaho; the rose, in Sarasota, Florida. A kaleidoscope, not shown, was added in Washington, D.C.

I was especially moved when a friend shared the story of her first tattoo:

My husband passed away in 2014 after a three-year journey with pancreatic cancer. While sick, he kept a blog and signed off each post with "All is Good." His positive attitude is what got me through that entire time. After he passed, I wanted to do something that would in some way mark me as having gone through that. My younger daughter came to me and said she wanted to have "All is good" tattooed on her ankle. I decided that was exactly what I wanted to do as well. Mine is in Hebrew and hers is in English.

She and her daughter are connected through their tattoos, just as the tattoos connect them with their husband and father.

They're not the only ones to use tattoos as a means of connection. Rachel Mashman wrote about how she and her daughter got matching tattoos on the first anniversary of her daughter's nearly successful suicide attempt. Getting the tattoos created a positive memory to replace the horror of the original day. They chose the image of an arrow, to represent strength, bravery, and moving forward. [3]

Once the hallmark of youth, low life, or wild behavior, tattoos have become mainstream and intergenerational, something you can do with and for others to create a meaningful shared experience. Tattoos can invite discourse and create opportunities to engage with others. They can connect us to those we have lost and to those who are still here. They can make us feel alive and current, even adventurous. Tattoos are so much more than ink.

Studies show that people who engage in meaningful, productive activities with others tend to have positive aging outcomes. They live longer, are happier, and have improved cognitive function and a sense of purpose. Conversely, social isolation and loneliness are associated with poor aging outcomes. The National Institute on Aging (NIA) is exploring potential interventions to reduce social isolation and loneliness.[4] Perhaps they should be looking at nail art.

Nail art is a way of embellishing nails with designs, artwork, glitter, patterns, and textures. For people of all ages, it's an opportunity for creativity, self-expression, and fun. It's also an opportunity for social interaction, and for some older people, nail art has been life-changing. After one eighty-seven-year-old woman was introduced to nail art, she began "hanging out" in the lobby of her senior-living community more than she used to, because people noticed her nails and would start conversations. Another woman in her eighties said nail art expressed her inner artistic side. Older women aren't supposed to be adventurous, spontaneous, frivolous, or outrageous, but aren't these part of what makes life exciting?

Studies show that people who engage in meaningful, productive activities with others tend to have positive aging outcomes.

The National Center for Creative Aging is dedicated to exploring the relationship between creative expression and quality of life of older people.[5] Nail art and tattoos are examples of creative expression, but they are also more than that. They are an opportunity for connection to others. We yearn for connection in every phase of our lives, especially as

Older women aren't supposed to be adventurous, spontaneous, frivolous, or outrageous, but aren't these part of what makes life exciting?

we age. Connection and creative expression as we age are within everyone's reach. They're at the tips of our fingers.

32

The Ten-Pound Mirror

It is sad to reach the end of a good book you are reading; you hate saying good-bye to the characters. I've discovered that it's sad reaching the end of a book you're writing, too. What note do you want to end on? What's the one thing you hope they'll take away? How do you, as the author, want to say good-bye?

I will say good-bye by telling you about our ten-pound mirror.

My husband and I have a ten-pound mirror. It's not that it weighs ten pounds. It's a floor-length mirror surrounded by engraved industrial wood. It's a work of art, really. But that's not why it's special. It's special because it's a ten-pound mirror.

There is something wrong with the optics. You walk by it, and then you come back and look at yourself again, and you look good—really good. Not totally different, just a little bit better than the real you. About ten pounds better.

We tend to be so hard on ourselves physically and emotionally. Maybe we need more ten-pound mirrors—a way to be more gentle with ourselves and our actions, less critical of how we look, more self-accepting . . . not because we are perfect, but because imperfection is *okay*. Maybe we all need our optics to be a little bit off.

Perhaps I am looking at this too narrowly. Maybe a ten-pound mirror doesn't have to be a thing. Perhaps it can be a person—someone who helps us see ourselves a little bit better than we really are. We might find a ten-pound mirror in a parent, a spouse, a sibling, a friend, even a child . . . someone who sees in us things we don't see ourselves, someone who sees us as the person we wish we were. And because of the image they reflect back to us, we see ourselves as a little bit better, too.

I know I have people in my life who have been ten-pound mirrors for me, and I am so very grateful. Their support, acceptance, and generosity have meant the world to me. I wonder if I have been a ten-pound mirror for someone else. I hope so.

Over the last few years, I've increasingly been asked, "Are you still working?", sometimes from people my age, sometimes from folks who are younger. It bothers me, because it feels as if there is more than curiosity behind the question; it feels like there is judgment.

Society seems to have preconceived notions of what we should be doing at a certain age, and I don't like being pigeon-holed into someone else's stereotype. I don't play tennis or mahjong. I am not part of a book group. I hate all things domestic. For a long time, I assumed I would not do well in retirement. I've read articles. Some suggest taking time—from several months to several years—to find your retirement purpose. Others say, "Don't retire from something, retire to something." This has appeal for me; I like being driven. I just need to find what I want to be driven by. That's why Encore.org speaks to me. [1] Encore.org was founded in 1998 by social entrepreneur Marc Freedman. Its goal is to redefine later life and shift the idea of retirement as freedom from work, to freedom to work and contribute in new ways and to new ends.

Encore focuses on the role of purpose in later life, and in 2005 created the Purpose Prize to honor social entrepreneurs over sixty who combine experience, purpose, and passion to make a difference in their communities and the world.[2] "It's not a lifetime achievement award," says Encore. "These folks are just getting started." Now that's a view of later life that appeals to me.

As I read stories of Purpose Prize honorees, I am humbled by their passion, determination, and accomplishment. These people refuse to accept the prevailing view of what later life is supposed to look like. Instead, they've created organizations and programs that empower others to work for a greater good.

I wish I could tell you that I've found my purpose. When I was working, I wanted my retirement purpose to be a quickly-arrived-at destination. So far, it's feeling more like a journey, and, to my surprise, I am valuing the time and experience. I've slowed down and am spending more time in the moment. I believe having purpose is important and that I'll eventually arrive at a destination, but I'm no longer impatient or worried. I am looking at life through a ten-pound mirror and life looks pretty good.

Squint Discussion Guide
and Book Club Kit

S quint is about situations people deal with every day. It invites discussion and is a great choice for book clubs.

Visit www.margitnovack.com to download a discussion guide with thought-provoking questions.

If you enjoyed *Squint*, I would be ever so grateful if you would write a review on my Amazon.com page.

—Margit Novack

Chapter Notes

Introduction

1. "In Praise of the Squint," The Painter's Keys, Robert Genn, http://painterskeys.com/praise-squint/
2. Founded in 1954, the American Society on Aging (ASA) is an association of diverse individuals committed to improving the quality of life of older adults and their families (http://www.asaging.org). The Business of the Year awards were given by the ASA's Business Forum on Aging.
3. "Moving A Lifetime" by Elizabeth Pope, Monday, June 21, 2004, http://content.time.com/time/magazine/article/0,9171,655420,00.html, https://www.nytimes.com/2005/04/12/business/retirement/their-specialty-anything-gray.html
4. www.nasmm.org. The National Association of Senior Move Managers (NASMM).
5. www.davidsolie.com, David Solie, *How To Say It To Seniors: Closing the Communication Gap with Our Elders.*

Chapter 1—Tough Love

1. https://consumer.healthday.com/mental-health-information-25/sedatives-health-news-598/1-in-4-seniors-who-take-xanax-valium-use-them-long-term-737573.html
2. The Charles C. Knox Home in Wynnewood, PA opened in 1941 as a non-sectarian independent living residence for older adults of modest means. It offered private rooms with shared baths and means in a common dining room, as well as other services. The home was closed in 2013.
3. https://www.nia.nih.gov/health/depression-and-older-adults
4. https://www.britannica.com/biography/Jack-Kevorkian

5. https://www.mayoclinicproceedings.org/article/S0025
-6196(16)30509-2/fulltext#%20, Benzodiazepine Use in Older
Adults: Dangers, Management and Alternative Therapies

Chapter 2—Medication Management

1. https://www.nps.org.au/australian-prescriber/articles/the
-prescribing-cascade
2. https://www.modernhealthcare.com/opinion-editorial
/fragmented-health-system-contributes-medication-overload
-seniors
3. https://academic.oup.com/psychsocgerontology/article/57/5
/P409/609413

Chapter 3—Technology Adoption

1. https://www.nia.nih.gov/health/hearing-loss-common-problem
-older-adults.
2. https://practicalneurology.com/articles/2017-oct/the-cognitive
-and-behavioral-consequences-of-hearing-loss-part-1

Chapter 4—Difficult Conversations

1. http://www.ellengoodman.com/, How to Talk About Dying,
by Ellen Goodman, *New York Times*, July 1, 2015
2. Additional resources for end-of-life discussions:
   • theconversationproject.org For resources on initiating end
   of life discussions with loved ones.
   • www.fivewishes.org For an easy-to-use advance directive
   document that speaks to all of a person's needs: medical,
   personal, emotional and spiritual.
   • www.mywonderfullife.com For information on how to plan
   and personalize your own funeral.

Chapter 5—The Importance of Being Needed

1. https://academic.oup.com/psychsocgerontology/article/62/1
/P28/572495, Feelings of Usefulness to Others, Disability, and
Mortality in Older Adults: The MacArthur Study of Successful
Aging

Chapter 8—Detaching With Love

1. https://www.agingcare.com/articles/setting-boundaries-with
   -parents-who-are-abusive-142804.htm, Detaching With Love:
   Setting Boundaries with Difficult Elderly Parents

Chapter 9—Senior Suicide

1. https://www.aamft.org/AAMFT/Consumer_Updates/Suicide
   _in_the_Elderly.aspx, American Association for Marriage and
   Family Therapy, Suicide in the Elderly
2. https://www.agingcare.com/articles/assisted-suicide-in-the
   -elderly-167708.htm, Assisted Suicide and Elders: How Far
   Would a Loving Caregiver Go?
3. https://www.griefincommon.com/blog/a-different-kind-of
   -loss-grieving-the-relationship-that-never-was/

Chapter 10—Sibling Estrangement

1. http://content.time.com/time/magazine/article/0,9171,91424
   ,00.html, Why We Break Up With Our Siblings by Lise Funderberg
2. https://www.psychologytoday.com/us/articles/201503/why
   -siblings-sever-ties, Why Siblings Sever Ties by Sara Eckel

Chapter 11—Personal Treasures

1. Downsizing: Confronting Our Possessions in Later Life Paper-
   back—June 16, 2020, Professor David Ekerdt

Chapter 12—Blended families

1. https://www.worldwidewords.org/qa/qa-red2.htm

Chapter 13—Forgiveness

1. https://www.asaging.org/blog/art-and-science-firegiveness,
   The Art and Science of Forgiveness, by Frederic Luskin
2. https://www.ncbi.nlm.nih.gov/pmc/articles/PMC2868276/
   Unforgiveness, Rumination, and Depressive Symptoms among
   Older Adults

Chapter 14—Letting Go of Ageism

1. https://iiasa.ac.at/web/home/research/researchPrograms /WorldPopulation/Reaging/Re-Aging.html Reassessing Aging From a Population Perspective
2. https://www.asaging.org/blog/history-ageism-1969, A History of Ageism Since 1969, W. Andrew Achenbaum
3. *Healthy Aging: A Lifelong Guide to Your Well-Being*, Andrew Weil, M.D.
4. https://www.hindawi.com/journals/jger/2015/954027/, Stereotypes of Aging: Their Effects on the Health of Older Adults, Rylee A. Dionigi

Chapter 15—Why My Purse Was in the Freezer

1. https://www.nia.nih.gov/health/what-are-signs-alzheimers -disease, What Are The Signs of Alzheimer's Disease?

Chapter 16—Mishearing

1. https://www.nia.nih.gov/health/hearing-loss-common-problem -older-adults, Senior Statistics

Chapter 17—Consumer Invisibility

1. https://www.pewresearch.org/internet/2017/05/17/technology -use-among-seniors/, Technology Use Among Seniors
2. https://www.acrwebsite.org/volumes/6307/volumes/v11 /NA-11, Buying and Consuming Behavior of the Elderly
3. https://www.aarp.org/content/dam/aarp/home-and-family /personal-technology/2013-10/Longevity-Economy-Generating -New-Growth-AARP.pdf, The Longevity Economy: Generating Economic Growth and New Opportunities for Business

Chapter 19—Diamonds in the Rough

1. https://girlshs.philasd.org/
2. https://time.com/4464811/aging-happiness-stress-anxiety-depression/, Older People are Happier Than People in Their Twenties
3. *I Feel Bad About My Neck: And Other Thoughts on Being a Woman*—2008, Nora Ephron

Part 4—Perfection Is Not Required

1. https://www.chron.com/life/houston-belief/article/Perlman
   -makes-his-music-the-hard-way-2009719.php, Perlman Makes
   His Music the Hard Way

Chapter 22—Fear of Abandonment

1. http://davidhilfiker.blogspot.com/2013/01/now-it-begins.html,
   Watching the Lights Go Out, A Memoir of an Uncertain Mind,
   David Hilfiker
2. *Four Funerals and a Wedding: Resilience in a Time of Grief*,
   Jill Smolowe

Chapter 23—Caregiving

1. https://psychcentral.com/lib/aging-parents-and-your-emotional
   -well-being/, Aging Parents and Your Emotional Well Being,
   Julie Axelrod.

Chapter 24—Plan B

1. https://www.presidency.ucsb.edu/documents/annual-message
   -the-congress-the-state-the-union-4

Chapter 25—Gifts with Strings

1. *Downsizing: Confronting Our Possessions in Later Life* Paper-
   back—June 16, 2020, Professor David Ekerdt

Chapter 26—The Ethics of Geriatric Fiblets

1. https://www.alternativesinalzheimerscare.com/the-art-of
   -utilizing-a-fiblet/
2. https://www.nasmm.org/about/ethics.cfm
3. https://www.bustle.com/p/telling-white-lies-is-associated-with
   -this-positive-trait-so-dont-beat-yourself-up-about-it-62658

Chapter 27—The Upside of Risk

1. https://changingaging.org/archives/safety-surplus-the-upside
   -of-risk/

2. https://www.agingcare.com/articles/benefits-of-elderly-own-ing-pets-113294.htm, The Healing Power of Pets for Seniors, Barbara Ballinger
3. https://www.nydailynews.com/new-york/collyer-brothers-brownstone-gallery-1.1187698, Inside the Collyer Brownstone: The Story of Harlem's Hermits and Their Hoarding
4. https://www.challengingdisorganization.org/clutter-hoarding-scale-

Part 5—Planting Trees

1. https://legacyproject.org/guides/whatislegacy.html What Is Legacy, Susan Bosak

Chapter 29—Creating Legacy

1. https://www.delconewsnetwork.com/countypress/news/harold-sampson-wants-to-make-the-world-a-little-better/article_503ef686-97d8-5e05-9c88-e4e7206b50bd.html
2. https://www.washingtonpost.com/archive/lifestyle/2001/04/07/a-measure-of-hope/0428485a-d25c-42f7-8690-2a9d7e70ebe0/, A Measure of Hope, Dale Smith
3. https://oneclipatatime.org/paper-clips-project/paper-clips-film/

Chapter 30—Creating Legacy Through Objects

1. https://extension.umn.edu/who-gets-grandmas-yellow-pie-platetm-workshop-facilitators-toolkit/who-gets-grandmas-yellow-pie-0

Chapter 31—The Art of Connection

1. https://seniorplanet.org/aging-with-attitude-inked-rebel-helen-lambin/
2. https://sixtyandme.com/tattoos-for-older-women-a-surprising-new-trend/
3. https://grownandflown.com/mother-daughter-tattoos/
4. https://www.nia.nih.gov/news/social-isolation-loneliness-older-people-pose-health-risks

5. https://uclartsandhealing.org/resources_pages/national-center
-for-creative-aging-ncca/

Chapter 33—The Ten-Pound Mirror

1. https://encore.org/
2. https://purposeprize.encore.org/

Acknowledgments

First and foremost, to my Moving Solutions team. You inspired and humbled me daily. You brought out the best in me. Together, we did work that mattered.

To Karen Reber and Pattison Hemmerly, for years my writing godmothers. Everything I wrote was better because you were involved.

To my NASMM colleagues, who believed in me and encouraged me to write this book.

To the American Society on Aging, for recognizing the importance of Senior Move Management so many years ago and for introducing me to the world of professionals in aging. You helped guide my path.

To Judy Gitenstein, who helped me discover the purpose for this book. I looked for an editor and found a friend.

To my family: Mark, Michael, Jason, Arwyn, Noah., Bill, Laura and Paul. Thank you for allowing me to share your stories.

To Anya, Bubbie, Aunt Betty, my mother and father. Writing about you filled holes in my heart.

To my clients, who taught me so many lessons about life and purpose. Serving you was an honor and a privilege.

To Bill, for supporting me in business and in life. I love you.

To Covid and to this book, you are both so intertwined. Covid provided enforced downtime during which the concept of this book percolated and evolved. The book provided much needed purpose during Covid. Amidst challenge and loss, I experienced growth and inspiration. Perhaps that is the lesson of this book.

About the Author

Margit (rhymes with target) Novack is an entrepreneur, thought leader and industry founder in Senior Move Management. She loves serving clients, managing her team and sharing with colleagues. After decades in the field of aging, she moved away from her life of work and title, to a new role—author, speaker, and champion of a re-visioned picture of aging. *Squint: Re-visioning the Second Half of Life*, is her first book.

Margit lives with her husband and three dogs (a retired Greyhound racer and two puppy mill rescues). She divides her time between Philadelphia, Pennsylvania and the eastern shore of Maryland, where she loves kayaking upwind. To learn more about Margit and *Squint*, please visit www.margitnovack.com.

Made in the USA
Middletown, DE
12 July 2021